Virtual Clinical Excursions—Medical-Surgical

for

Monahan/Sands/Neighbors/Marek/Green
Phipps' Medical-Surgical Nursing:
Health and Illness Perspectives,
8th Edition

Virtual Clinical Excursions—Medical-Surgical

for

Monahan/Sands/Neighbors/Marek/Green
Phipps' Medical-Surgical Nursing:
Health and Illness Perspectives,
8th Edition

prepared by

Dorothy Mathers, RN, MSN
Associate Professor, Nursing
Pennsylvania College of Technology
Williamsport, Pennsylvania

software developed by

Wolfsong Informatics, LLC
Tucson, Arizona

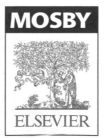

Contents

Unit 8—Endocrine Problems

Unit 9—Gastrointestinal Problems

Unit 10—Musculoskeletal Problems

Unit 11—Eye Problems

Table of Contents
Monahan/Sands/Neighbors/Marek/Green
Phipps' Medical-Surgical Nursing:
Health and Illness Perspectives, 8th Edition

■ INSTALLATION INSTRUCTIONS

WINDOWS

1. Insert the *Virtual Clinical Excursion—Medical-Surgical* CD-ROM.
2. Inserting the CD should automatically bring up the setup screen if the current product is not already installed.
   a. If the setup screen does not appear automatically (and *Virtual Clinical Excursion—Medical-Surgical* has not been installed already), navigate to the "My Computer" icon on your desktop or in your Start menu.
   b. Double-click on your CD-ROM drive.
   c. If installation does not start at this point:
      (1) Click the **Start** icon on the task bar and select the **Run** option.
      (2) Type d:\setup.exe (where "d:\" is your CD-ROM drive) and press **OK**.
      (3) Follow the onscreen instructions for installation.
3. Follow the onscreen instructions during the setup process.

MACINTOSH

1. Insert the *Virtual Clinical Excursion—Medical-Surgical* CD in the CD-ROM drive. The disk icon will appear on your desktop.

2. Double-click on the disk icon.

3. Double-click on the MEDICAL-SURGICAL_MAC run file.

NOTE: *Virtual Clinical Excursion—Medical-Surgical* for Macintosh does not have an installation setup and can only be run directly from the CD.

■ HOW TO USE VIRTUAL CLINICAL EXCURSIONS—MEDICAL-SURGICAL

WINDOWS

1. Double-click on the *Virtual Clinical Excursion—Medical-Surgical* icon located on your desktop.
2. Or navigate to the program via the Windows Start menu.

NOTE: Windows 98/ME will require you to restart your computer before running the *Virtual Clinical Excursion—Medical-Surgical* program.

MACINTOSH

1. Insert the *Virtual Clinical Excursion—Medical-Surgical* CD in the CD-ROM drive. The disk icon will appear on your desktop.

2. Double-click on the disk icon.

3. Double-click on the MEDICAL-SURGICAL_MAC run file.

■ SCREEN SETTINGS

For best results, your computer monitor resolution should be set at a minimum of 800 x 600. The number of colors displayed should be set to "thousands or higher" (High Color or 16 bit) or "millions of colors" (True Color or 24 bit).

Windows™

1. From the **Start** menu, select **Control Panel** (on some systems, you will first go to **Settings**, then to **Control Panel**).
2. Double-click on the **Display** icon.
3. Click on the **Settings** tab.
4. Under **Screen resolution** use the slider bar to select **800 by 600 pixels**.
5. Access the **Colors** drop-down menu by clicking on the down arrow.
6. Select **High Color (16 bit)** or **True Color (24 bit)**.
7. Click on **OK**.
8. You may be asked to verify the setting changes. Click **Yes**.
9. You may be asked to restart your computer to accept the changes. Click **Yes**.

Macintosh®

1. Select the **Monitors** control panel.
2. Select **800 x 600** (or similar) from the **Resolution** area.
3. Select **Thousands** or **Millions** from the **Color Depth** area.

■ WEB BROWSERS

Supported web browsers include Microsoft Internet Explorer (IE) version 6.0 or higher, Netscape version 7.1 or higher, and Mozilla Firefox.

If you use America Online (AOL) for web access, you will need AOL version 4.0 or higher and one of the browsers listed above. Do not use earlier versions of AOL with earlier versions of IE, because you will have difficulty accessing many features.

For best results with AOL:
* Connect to the Internet using AOL version 4.0 or higher.
* Open a private chat within AOL (this allows the AOL client to remain open, without asking whether you wish to disconnect while minimized).
* Minimize AOL.
* Launch a recommended browser.

■ TECHNICAL SUPPORT

Technical support for this product is available between 7:30 a.m. and 7 p.m. CST, Monday through Friday. Before calling, be sure that your computer meets the minimum system requirements to run this software. Inside the United States and Canada, call 1-800-692-9010. Outside North America, call 314-872-8370. You may also fax your questions to 314-523-4932 or contact Technical Support through e-mail: technical.support@elsevier.com.

Trademarks: Windows, Macintosh, Pentium, and America Online are registered trademarks.

Copyright © 2007 by Mosby, Inc., an affiliate of Elsevier Inc.

All rights reserved. No part of this product may be reproduced or transmitted in any form or by any means, electronic or mechanical, including input or storage in any information system, without written permission from the publisher.

ACCESSING *Virtual Clinical Excursions—Medical-Surgical* FROM EVOLVE ─────────────

The product you have purchased is part of the Evolve family of online courses and learning resources. Please read the following information completely to get started.

To access your instructor's course on Evolve:

Your instructor will provide you with the username and password needed to access their specific course on the Evolve Learning System. Once you have received this information, please follow these instructions:

1. Go to the Evolve student page (http://evolve.elsevier.com/student)

2. Enter your username and password in the **Login to My Evolve** area and click the **Login** button.

3. You will be taken to your personalized **My Evolve** page where the course will be listed in the **My Courses** module.

TECHNICAL REQUIREMENTS

To use an Evolve course, you will need access to a computer that is connected to the Internet and equipped with web browser software that supports frames. For optimal performance, it is recommended that you have speakers and use a high-speed Internet connection. However, slower dial-up modems (56 K minimum) are acceptable.

Whichever browser you use, the browser preferences must be set to enable cookies and Java/JavaScript and the cache must be set to reload every time.

Enable Cookies

Browser	Steps
Internet Explorer (IE) 6.0 or higher	1. Select **Tools**. 2. Select **Internet Options**. 3. Select **Privacy** tab. 4. Use the slider (slide down) to **Accept All Cookies**. 5. Click **OK**. -OR- 4. Click the **Advanced** button. 5. Click the check box next to **Override Automatic Cookie Handling**. 6. Click the **Accept** buttons under **First-party Cookies** and **Third-party Cookies**. 7. Click **OK**.
Netscape 7.1 or higher	1. Select **Edit**. 2. Select **Preferences**. 3. Select **Privacy & Security**. 4. Select **Cookies**. 5. Select **Enable All Cookies**.
Mozilla Firefox	1. Select **Tools → Options**. 2. Select the **Privacy** icon. 3. Click to expand Cookies. 4. Select **Allow sites to set cookies**. 5. Click **OK**.

Enable Java

Browser	Steps
Internet Explorer (IE) 6.0 or higher	1. Select **Tools → Internet Options**. 2. Select **Advanced** tab. 3. Scroll down the list until you see the **Java (Sun)** section and select the box that appears below it.
Netscape 7.1 or higher	1. Select **Edit → Preferences**. 2. Select **Advanced**. 3. Select **Scripts & Plugins**. 4. Make sure the **Navigator** box is checked to **Enable JavaScript**. 5. Click **OK**.
Mozilla Firefox	1. Select **Tools → Options**. 2. Select the **Web Features** icon. 3. Select **Enable Java**. 4. Select **Enable JavaScript**. 5. Click **OK**.

Set Cache to Always Reload a Page

Browser	Steps
Internet Explorer (IE) 6.0 or higher	1. Select **Tools → Internet Options**. 2. Select **General** tab. 3. Go to the **Temporary Internet Files** and click the **Settings** button. 4. Select the radio button for **Every visit to the page** and click **OK** when complete.
Netscape 7.1 or higher	1. Select **Edit → Preferences**. 2. Select **Advanced**. 3. Select **Cache**. 4. Select the **Every time I view the page** radio button. 5. Click **OK**.
Mozilla Firefox	1. Select **Tools → Options**. 2. Select the **Privacy** icon. 3. Click to expand Cache. 4. Set the value to "0" in the **Use up to: KB of disk space for the cache** field. 5. Click **OK**.

Plug-Ins

Adobe Acrobat Reader—With the free Acrobat Reader software you can view and print Adobe PDF files. Many Evolve products offer student and instructor manuals, checklists, and more in this format!

Download at: *http://www.adobe.com*

Apple QuickTime—Install this to hear word pronunciations, heart and lung sounds, and many other helpful audio clips within Evolve Online Courses!

Download at: *http://www.apple.com*

Macromedia Flash Player—This player will enhance your viewing of many Evolve web pages, as well as educational short-form to long-form animation within the Evolve Learning System!

Download at: *http://www.macromedia.com*

Macromedia Shockwave Player—Shockwave is best for viewing the many interactive learning activities within Evolve Online Courses!

Download at: *http://www.macromedia.com*

Microsoft Word Viewer—With this viewer Microsoft Word users can share documents with those who don't have Word, and users without Word can open and view Word documents. Many Evolve products have testbank, student and instructor manuals, and other documents available for downloading and viewing on your own computer!

Download at: *http://www.microsoft.com*

Microsoft PowerPoint Viewer—View PowerPoint 97, 2000, and 2002 presentations even if you don't have PowerPoint with this viewer. Many Evolve products have slides available for downloading and viewing on your own computer!

Download at: *http://www.microsoft.com*

SUPPORT INFORMATION

Live support is available to customers in the United States and Canada from 7:30 a.m. to 7:00 p.m. (Central Time), Monday through Friday by calling, **1-800-401-9962**. You can also send an email to evolve-support@elsevier.com.

There is also **24/7 support information** available on the Evolve website (http://evolve.elsevier.com), including:

- Guided Tours
- Tutorials
- Frequently Asked Questions (FAQs)
- Online Copies of Course User Guides
- And much more!

A QUICK TOUR

Welcome to *Virtual Clinical Excursions—Medical-Surgical*, a virtual hospital setting in which you can work with multiple complex patient simulations and also learn to access and evaluate the information resources that are essential for high-quality patient care.

The virtual hospital, Pacific View Regional Hospital, has realistic architecture and access to patient rooms, a Nurses' Station, and a Medication Room.

■ BEFORE YOU START

Make sure you have your textbook nearby when you use the *Virtual Clinical Excursions—Medical-Surgical* CD. You will want to consult topic areas in your textbook frequently while working with the CD and using this workbook.

■ HOW TO SIGN IN

- Enter your name on the Student Nurse identification badge.
- Now click the down arrow next to **Select Period of Care**. This drop-down menu gives you four periods of care from which to choose. In Periods of Care 1 through 3, you can actively engage in patient assessment, entry of data in the electronic patient record (EPR), and medication administration. Period of Care 4 presents the day in review. Highlight and click the appropriate period of care. (For this quick tour, choose **Period of Care 2**.)
- Click **Go** in the lower right side of the screen.
- This takes you to the Patient List screen (see example on page 11). Only the patients on the floor you choose (Medical-Surgical) are available. Note that the virtual time is provided in the box at the lower left corner of the screen (1115, since we chose Period of Care 2).

Note: If you choose to work during Period of Care 4: 1900-2000, the Patient List screen is skipped since you are not able to visit patients or administer medications during the shift. Instead, you are taken directly to the Nurses' Station, where the records of all the patients on the floor are available for your review.

■ **PATIENT LIST**

MEDICAL-SURGICAL UNIT

Harry George (Room 401)
Osteomyelitis—A middle-aged Caucasian male admitted from a homeless shelter with an infected leg. He has complications of type 2 diabetes mellitus, alcohol abuse, nicotine addiction, poor pain control, and complex psychosocial issues.

Jacquline Catanazaro (Room 402)
Asthma—A middle-aged Caucasian female admitted with an acute asthma exacerbation and suspected pneumonia. She has complications of chronic schizophrenia, noncompliance with medication therapy, obesity, and herniated disc.

Piya Jordan (Room 403)
Bowel obstruction—An older Asian female admitted with a colon mass and suspected adenocarcinoma. She undergoes a right hemicolectomy. This patient's complications include atrial fibrillation, hypokalemia, and symptoms of meperidine toxicity.

Clarence Hughes (Room 404)
Degenerative joint disease—An older African-American male admitted for a left total knee replacement. His preparations for discharge are complicated by the development of a pulmonary embolus and the need for ongoing intravenous therapy.

Pablo Rodriguez (Room 405)
Metastatic lung carcinoma—An older Hispanic male admitted with symptoms of dehydration and malnutrition. He has chronic pain secondary to multiple subcutaneous skin nodules and psychosocial concerns related to family issues with his approaching death.

Patricia Newman (Room 406)
Pneumonia—A middle-aged female admitted with worsening pulmonary function and an acute respiratory infection. Her chronic emphysema is complicated by heavy smoking, hypertension, and malnutrition. She needs access to community resources such as a smoking cessation program and meal assistance.

■ HOW TO SELECT A PATIENT

- You can choose one or more patients to work with from the Patient List by clicking the box to the left of the patient name(s). (In order to receive a scorecard for a patient, the patient must be selected before proceeding to the Nurses' Station.)
- Click on **Get Report** to the right of the medical records number (MRN) to view a summary of the patient's care during the 12-hour period before your arrival on the unit.
- When you are ready to begin your care, click on **Go to Nurses' Station** in the right lower corner.

Virtual Clinical Excursions 3.0 : Medical Surgical Patient Set

Patient List

	Patient Name	Room	MRN	Clinical Report
☐	Harry George	401	1868054	Get Report
☐	Jacquline Catanazaro	402	1868048	Get Report
☑	Piya Jordan	403	1868092	Get Report
☐	Clarence Hughes	404	1868011	Get Report
☑	Pablo Rodriguez	405	1868088	Get Report
☐	Patricia Newman	406	1868097	Get Report

Please select all the patients you will be caring for this period of care. Once you have exited the patient list, you will not be able to change your current selections or select new patients to care for.

0730   Go to Nurses' Station

■ HOW TO FIND A PATIENT'S RECORDS

NURSES' STATION

Within the Nurses' Station, you will see:

1. A clipboard that contains the patient list for that floor.
2. A chart rack with patient charts labeled by room number, a notebook labeled Kardex, and a notebook labeled MAR (Medication Administration Record).
3. A desktop computer with access to the Electronic Patient Record (EPR).
4. A tool bar across the top of the screen that can also be used to access the Patient List, EPR, Chart, MAR, and Kardex. This tool bar is also accessible from each patient's room.
5. A Drug Guide containing information about the medications you are able to administer to your patients.

As you run your cursor over an item, it will be highlighted. To select, simply double-click on the item. As you use these resources, you will always be able to return to the Nurses' Station by clicking on the **Return to Nurses' Station** bar located in the right lower corner of your screen.

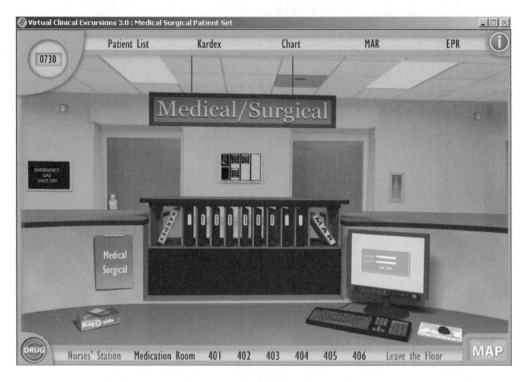

MEDICATION ADMINISTRATION RECORD (MAR)

The MAR icon located in the tool bar at the top of your screen accesses current 24-hour medications for each patient. Click on the icon and the MAR will open. (*Note:* You can also access the MAR by clicking on the blue MAR notebook on the far right side of the book rack in the center of the screen.) Within the MAR, tabs on the right side of the screen allow you to select patients by room number. Be careful to make sure you select the correct tab number for *your* patient rather than simply reading the first record that appears after the MAR opens. Each MAR sheet lists the following:

- Medications
- Route and dosage of medications
- Times of administration of medication

Note: The MAR changes each day. Expired MARs are stored in the patients' charts.

CHARTS

To access patient charts, either click on the **Chart** icon at the top of your screen or anywhere within the chart rack in the center of the Nurses' Station screen. When the close-up view appears, the individual charts are labeled by room number. To open a chart, click on the room number of the patient whose chart you wish to review. The patient's name and allergies will appear, along with a list of tabs on the right side of the screen, allowing you to view the following data:

- Allergies
- Physician's Orders
- Physician's Notes
- Nurse's Notes
- Laboratory Reports
- Diagnostic Reports
- Surgical Reports
- Consultations

- Patient Education
- History and Physical
- Nursing Admission
- Expired MARs
- Consents
- Mental Health
- Admissions
- Emergency Department

Information appears in real time. The entries are in reverse chronological order, so use the down arrow at the right side of the chart page to scroll down to view previous entries. Flip from tab to tab to view multiple data fields or click on the **Return to Nurses' Station** bar in the lower right corner of the screen to exit the chart.

ELECTRONIC PATIENT RECORD (EPR)

The EPR can be accessed from the computer in the Nurses' Station or from the EPR icon located in the tool bar at the top of your screen. To access a patient's EPR:
- Click on either the computer screen or the **EPR** icon.
- Your user name and password are automatically filled in.
- Click on **Login** to enter the EPR.

The EPR used in Pacific View Regional Hospital represents a composite of commercial versions being used in hospitals. You can access the EPR:
- for a patient (by room number).
- to review existing data.
- to enter data you collect while working with a patient.

The EPR is updated daily, so no matter what day or part of a shift you are working, there will be a current EPR with the patient's data from the past days of the current hospital stay. This type of simulated EPR allows you to examine how data for different attributes have changed over time, as well as to examine data for all of a patient's attributes at a particular time. The EPR is fully functional (as it is in a real-life hospital). You can enter such data as blood pressure, breath sounds, and certain treatments. The EPR will not, however, allow you to enter data for a previous time period. Use the arrows at the bottom of the screen to move forward and backward in time.

Virtual Clinical Excursions 3.0 : Medical Surgical Patient Set				
Patient: 403 Category: Vital Signs				0732
Name: Piya Jordan	Wed 0630	Wed 0700	Wed 0715	Code Meanings
PAIN: LOCATION		OS		A — Abdomen
PAIN: RATING		5		Ar — Arm
PAIN: CHARACTERISTICS		C		B — Back
PAIN: VOCAL CUES		VC3		C — Chest
PAIN: FACIAL CUES		FC1		Ft — Foot
PAIN: BODILY CUES				H — Head
PAIN: SYSTEM CUES				Hd — Hand
PAIN: FUNCTIONAL EFFECTS				L — Left
PAIN: PREDISPOSING FACTORS				Lg — Leg
PAIN: RELIEVING FACTORS				Lw — Lower
PCA		P		N — Neck
TEMPERATURE (F)		99.6		NN — See Nurses notes
TEMPERATURE (C)				OS — Operative site
MODE OF MEASUREMENT		Ty		Or — See Physicians orders
SYSTOLIC PRESSURE		110		PN — See Progress notes
DIASTOLIC PRESSURE		70		R — Right
BP MODE OF MEASUREMENT		NIBP		Up — Upper
HEART RATE		104		
RESPIRATORY RATE		18		
SpO2 (%)		95		
BLOOD GLUCOSE				
WEIGHT				
HEIGHT				
◀		▮▷		Exit EPR

At the top of the EPR screen, you can choose patients by their room numbers. In addition, you have access to 17 different categories of patient data. To change patients or data categories, click the down arrow to the right of the room number or category.

The categories of patient data in the EPR as as follows:

- Vital Signs
- Respiratory
- Cardiovascular
- Neurologic
- Gastrointestinal
- Excretory
- Musculoskeletal
- Integumentary
- Reproductive
- Psychosocial
- Wounds and Drains
- Activity
- Hygiene and Comfort
- Safety
- Nutrition
- IV
- Intake and Output

Remember, each hospital selects its own codes. The codes used in the EPR at Pacific View Regional Hospital may be different from ones you have seen in clinical rotations that have computerized patient records. Take some time to acquaint yourself with the codes. Within the Vital Signs category, click on any item in the left column (e.g., heart rate). In the far-right column, you will see a list of code meanings for the possible findings and/or descriptors for that assessment area.

You will use the codes to record the data you collect as you work with patients. Click on the box in the last time column to the right of the data and wait for the code meanings applicable to that entry to appear. Select the appropriate code to describe your assessment findings and type it in the box. (*Note:* If no cursor appears within the box, click on the box again until the blue shading disappears and the blinking cursor appears.) Once the data are typed in this box, they are entered into the patient's record for this period of care only.

To leave the EPR, click on **Exit EPR** in the bottom right corner of the screen.

■ VISITING A PATIENT

From the Nurses' Station, click on the room number of the patient you wish to visit in the tool bar at the bottom of your screen. Once you are inside the room, you will see a still photo of your patient in the top left corner. To verify that this is the patient you have chosen, click on the **Check Armband** icon to the right of the photo. The patient's identification data will appear. If you click on **Check Allergies** (the next icon to the right), a list of the patient's allergies (if any) will replace the photo.

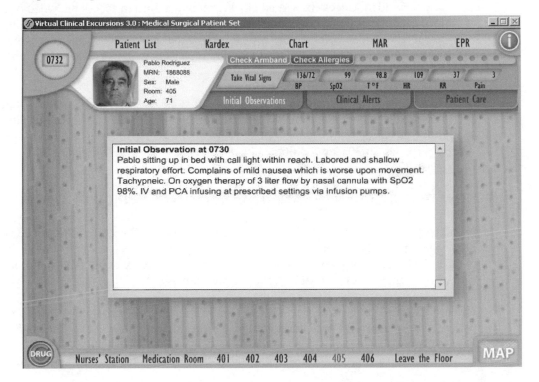

Also located in the patient's room are multiple icons you may use to assess the patient or the patient's medications. A clock is provided in the upper left corner of the room to monitor your progress in real time.

- The tool bar across the top of the screen allows you to check the **Patient List**, access the **EPR** to check or enter data, and view the patient's **Chart**, **MAR**, or **Kardex**.

- The **Take Vital Signs** icon allows you to measure the patient's up-to-the-minute blood pressure, oxygen saturation, temperature, heart rate, respiratory rate, and pain level.

- When you click on **Initial Observations**, a description appears in the text box under the patient's photo, allowing you a "look" at the patient as if you had just stepped in. To the right of this icon is **Clinical Alerts**, a resource that allows you to make decisions about priority medication interventions based on emerging data collected in real time. Check this screen throughout your period of care to avoid missing critical information related to recently ordered or STAT medications.

- Clicking on the **Patient Care** icon opens up three specific learning environments within the patient room: **Physical Assessment**, **Nurse-Client Interactions**, and **Medication Administration**.

- To perform a **Physical Assessment**, choose a body area (such as **Head & Neck**) by clicking on the appropriate icon in the column of yellow buttons. This activates a list of system subcategories for that body area (e.g., see **Sensory**, **Neurologic**, etc. in the green boxes). After you click on the system that you wish to evaluate, a still photo and text box appear, describing the assessment findings. The still photo is a "snapshot" of how an assessment of this area might be done or what the finding might look like. For every body area, there is also an **Equipment** button located on the far right of the screen.

- To the right of the Physical Assessment icon is **Nurse-Client Interactions**. Clicking on this icon will reveal the times and titles of any videos available for viewing. (*Note:* If the video you wish to see is not listed, this means you have not yet reached the correct virtual time to view that video. Check the virtual clock; you may return to access the video once its designated time has occurred—as long as you do so within the corresponding period of care.) To view a listed video, click on the white arrow to the right of the video title. Use the square control buttons below the video to start, stop, pause, rewind, or fast-forward the action or to mute the sound.

- **Medication Administration** is the pathway that allows you to review and administer medications to a patient after you have prepared them in the Medication Room. This process is addressed further in the *How to Prepare Medications* section (pages 19-20) and in *Medications* (pages 26-30). For additional hands-on practice, see *Reducing Medication Errors* (pages 37-41).

■ HOW TO QUIT, CHANGE PATIENTS, OR CHANGE PERIOD OF CARE

How to Quit: From most screens, you may click the **Leave the Floor** icon on the bottom tool bar to the right of the patient room numbers. (*Note:* From some screens, you will first need to click an **Exit** button or **Return to Nurses' Station** before clicking **Leave the Floor**.) When the Floor Menu appears, click **Exit** to leave the program.

How to Change Patients or Period of Care: To change patients, simply click on the new patient's room number. (You cannot receive a scorecard for a new patient, however, unless you have already selected that patient on the Patient List screen.) To change to a new period of care or restart the virtual clock for a new patient, click the **Leave the Floor** icon and then **Restart**.

Floor Menu screen (Virtual Clinical Excursions 3.0 : Medical Surgical Patient Set)

- Look at your Preceptor's Evaluation.
  Evaluations provide feedback on the work you completed during patient care. If you choose the Preceptor's Evaluation you will no longer be able to return to the floor.
- Take a break.
  Time will be stopped until you wish to return to the simulation.
- Restart the program.
  If you restart, all data from your work in the current Period of Care will be erased.
- View Credits
  Take a look at the list of professionals who took part in the creation of this software suite.
- Exit the program.
  If you choose to exit, all data from your work within the current Period of Care will be erased.

0732   Return to Room 405

■ HOW TO PREPARE MEDICATIONS

From the Nurses' Station or the patient's room, you can access the Medication Room by clicking on the icon in the tool bar at the bottom of your screen to the left of the patient room numbers.

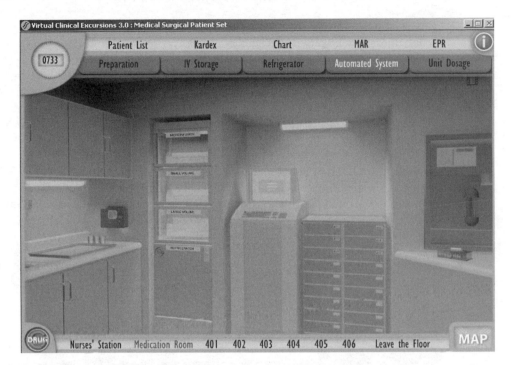

In the Medication Room you have access to the following (from left to right):

- A preparation area is located on the counter under the cabinets. To begin the medication preparation process, click on the tray on the counter or click on the **Preparation** icon at the top of the screen. The next screen leads you through a preparation sequence (called the Preparation Wizard) to prepare medications one at a time for administration to a patient. However, no medication has been selected at this time. We will do this while working with a patient in *A Detailed Tour*. To exit this screen, click on **View the Medication Room**.

- To the right of the cabinets (and above the refrigerator), IV storage bins are provided. Click on the bins themselves or on the **IV Storage** icon at the top of the screen. The bins are labeled **Microinfusion**, **Small Volume**, and **Large Volume**. Click on an individual bin to see a list of its contents. No medications are available in the bins at this time, but if they were, you could click on an individual medication and its label would appear to the right under the patient's name. Next, you would click **Put Medication on Tray**. If you ever change your mind or choose the incorrect medication, you can reverse your actions by clicking on **Put Medication in Bin**. Click **Close Bin** in the right bottom corner to exit. **View Medication Room** brings you back to a full view of the entire room.

- A refrigerator is located under the IV storage bins to hold any medications that must be stored below room temperature. Click on it to remove your medications; then click **Close Door**. You can also access this area by clicking the **Refrigerator** icon at the top of the screen.

- To prepare controlled substances, click the **Automated System** icon at the top of the screen or click the computer monitor located to the right of the IV storage bins. A login screen will appear; your name and password are automatically filled in. Click **Login**. Select a patient to log medications out for; then select the drawer you wish to open. Click **Open Drawer**, choose **Put Medication on Tray**, and then click **Close Drawer**.

- Next to the Automated System is a set of drawers identified by patient room number. To access these, click on the drawers themselves or on the **Unit Dosage** icon at the top of the screen. This provides a close-up view of the drawers. Click on the room number of the patient you are working with to open that drawer. Next, click on the medication you would like to prepare for the patient, and a label appears to the right under the patient's name, listing strength, units, and dosage per unit. You can **Open** and **Close** this medication label by clicking the appropriate icon. To exit, click **Close Drawer**; then click **View Medication Room**.

At any time, you can learn about a medication you wish to prepare for a patient by clicking on the **Drug** icon in the bottom left corner of the medication room screen or by clicking the **Drug Guide** book on the counter to the right of the unit dosage drawers. The **Drug Guide** provides information about the medications commonly included in nursing drug handbooks. Nutritional supplements and maintenance intravenous fluid preparations are not included.

To access the MAR to review the medications ordered for a patient, click on the **MAR** icon located in the tool bar at the top of your screen. You may also click the **Review MAR** icon in the tool bar at the bottom of your screen from inside each medication storage area.

After you have chosen and prepared your medications, return to the patient's room to administer them by clicking on the room number in the bottom tool bar. Once inside the patient's room, click on **Medication Administration** and follow the administration sequence.

■ PRECEPTOR'S EVALUATIONS

When you have finished a session, click on **Leave the Floor** to go to the Floor Menu. At this point, you can click on the icon next to **Look at your Preceptor's Evaluation** to receive a scorecard that provides feedback on the work you completed during patient care.

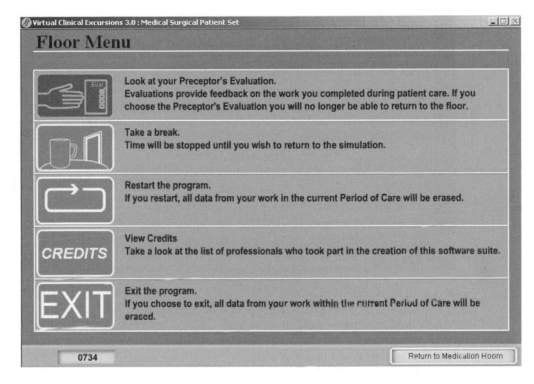

Evaluations are available for each patient you signed in for. Click on any of the **Medication Scorecard** icons to see an example. The scorecard compares the medications you administered to a patient during a period of care with what should have been administered. Table A lists the correct medications. Table B lists any medications that were administered incorrectly.

A DETAILED TOUR

If you wish to more thoroughly understand the capabilities of *Virtual Clinical Excursions—Medical-Surgical*, take a detailed tour by completing the following section. During this tour, we will work with a specific patient to introduce you to all the different components and learning opportunities available within the software.

■ WORKING WITH A PATIENT

Sign in and select the Medical-Surgical floor for Period of Care 1 (0730-0815). From the Patient List, select Piya Jordan in Room 403; however, do not go to the Nurses' Station yet.

Virtual Clinical Excursions 3.0 : Medical Surgical Patient Set

Patient List

	Patient Name	Room	MRN	Clinical Report
☐	Harry George	401	1868054	Get Report
☐	Jacquline Catanazaro	402	1868048	Get Report
☑	Piya Jordan	403	1868092	Get Report
☐	Clarence Hughes	404	1868011	Get Report
☑	Pablo Rodriguez	405	1868088	Get Report
☐	Patricia Newman	406	1868097	Get Report

0730   Return to Nurses' Station

■ REPORT

In hospitals, when one shift ends and another begins, the outgoing nurse who attended a patient will give a verbal and sometimes a written summary of that patient's condition to the incoming nurse who will assume care for the patient. This summary is called a report and is an important source of data to provide an overview of a patient. Your first task is to get clinical report on Piya Jordan. To do this, click **Get Report** in the far right column in this patient's row. From this summary, identify the problems and areas of concern that you will need to address for this patient.

When you have finished reading the report and noting any areas of concern, click **Go to Nurses' Station**.

■ CHARTS

You can access Piya Jordan's chart from the Nurses' Station or from the patient's room (403). We will access it from the Nurses' Station: Click on the chart rack or on the **Chart** icon in the tool bar at the top of your screen. Next, click on the chart labeled **403** to open the medical record for Piya Jordan. Click on the **Emergency Department** tab to view a record of why this patient was admitted.

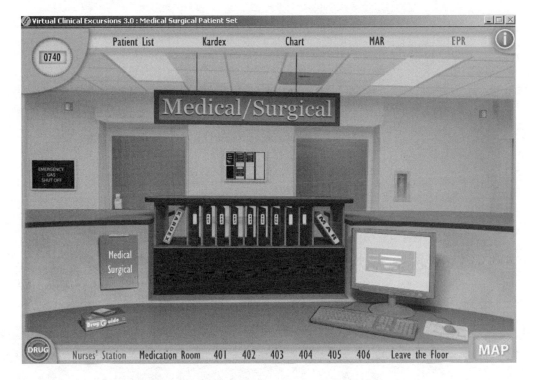

How many days has Piya Jordan been in the hospital?

What tests were done upon her arrival in the Emergency Department and why?

What was her reason for admission?

You should also click on **Surgical Reports** to learn what procedures were performed and when. Finally, review the **Nursing Admission** and **History and Physical** tabs to view information on the health history of this patient. When you are done reviewing the chart, click **Return to Nurses' Station**.

■ MEDICATIONS

Open the Medication Administration Record (MAR) by clicking on the **MAR** icon in the tool bar at the top of your screen. *Remember:* The MAR automatically opens to the first occupied room number on the floor (in this case, Room 401, Harry George). Since you need to access Piya Jordan's MAR, click on tab **403** (her room number). Always make sure you are giving the *Right Drug to the Right Patient!*

Examine the list of medications prescribed for Piya Jordan. Write down the medications that need to be given during this period of care (0730-0815). For each medication, note the dosage, route, and time in the chart below.

Time	Medication	Dosage	Route
0800	Digoxin	0.125 mg	IV

Click on **Return to Nurses' Station**. Next, click on **403** on the bottom tool bar and then verify that you are indeed in Piya Jordan's room. Select **Clinical Alerts** (the icon to the right of Initial Observations) to check for any emerging data that might affect your medication administration priorities. Go to the patient's chart (click on the **Chart** icon; then click on **403**). When the chart opens, select the **Physician's Orders** tab.

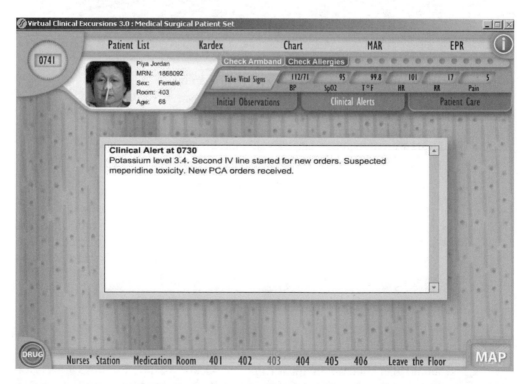

Review the orders. Have any new medications been ordered? Return to the MAR (click **Return to Room 403**; then click **MAR**). Verify that the new medications have been correctly transcribed to the MAR. Mistakes are sometimes made in the transcription process in the hospital setting, and it is sound practice to double-check any new order.

Are there any patient assessments you will need to perform before administering these medications? If so, return to Room 403 and click on **Patient Care** and then **Physical Assessment** to complete those before proceeding. (*Hint:* Check apical pulse.)

Now click on the **Medication Room** icon in the tool bar at the bottom of your screen to locate and prepare the medications for Piya Jordan.

In the Medication Room, you must access the medications for Piya Jordan from the specific dispensing system in which each medication is stored. Locate each medication that needs to be given in this time period and click on **Put Medication on Tray** as appropriate. (*Hint:* Look in Unit Dosage drawer first.) When you are finished, click on **Close Drawer** and then on **View Medication Room**. Now click on the medication tray on the counter on the left side of the medication room screen to begin preparing the medications you have selected. (*Note:* Instead of clicking on the tray, you can click **Preparation** at top of screen.)

In the preparation area, you should see a list of the medications you put on the tray in the previous steps. Click on the first medication and then click **Prepare**. Follow the onscreen instructions of the Preparation Wizard, providing any data requested. As an example, let's follow the preparation process for digoxin, one of the medications due to be administered to Piya Jordan during this period of care. To begin, click to select **Digoxin**; then click **Prepare**. Now work through the Preparation Wizard sequence as detailed below:

Amount of medication in the ampule: 2 mL
Enter the amount of medication you will draw up into a syringe: **0.5** mL
Click **Next**.
Select the patient you wish to set aside the medication for:
Click **Room 403, Piya Jordan**.
Click **Finish**.
Click **Return to Medication Room**.

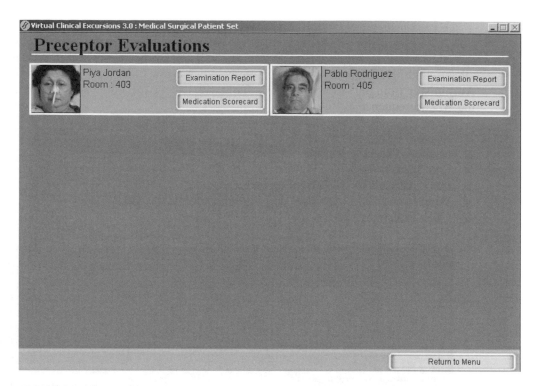

MEDICATION SCORECARD

- First, review Table A. Was digoxin given correctly? Did you give the other medications as ordered?
- Table B shows you which (if any) medications you gave incorrectly.
- Table C addresses the resources used for Piya Jordan. Did you access the patient's chart, MAR, EPR, or Kardex as needed to make safe medication administration decisions?
- Did you check the patient's armband to verify her identity? Did you check whether your patient had any known allergies to medications? Were vital signs taken?

Now that you understand the basic steps of medication preparation and administration, the following section will allow you to practice these skills further—with an increased emphasis on reducing medication errors by using the Medication Scorecard to evaluate your work.

■ VITAL SIGNS

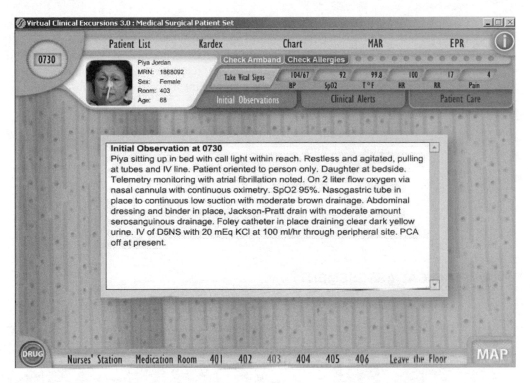

Vital signs, often considered the traditional signs of life, include body temperature, heart rate, respiratory rate, blood pressure, oxygen saturation of the blood, and the patient's experience of pain.

Inside Piya Jordan's room, click **Take Vital Signs**. (*Remember:* You can take vital signs at any time. The data change over time to reflect the temporal changes you would find in a patient similar to Piya Jordan.) Collect vital signs for this patient and record them in the following table. Note the time at which you collected each of these data.

Vital Signs	Findings/Time
Blood pressure	
O$_2$ saturation	
Heart rate	
Respiratory rate	
Temperature	
Pain rating	

After you are done, click on the **EPR** icon located in the tool bar at the top of the screen.

Complete the EPR Login screen as directed in *A Quick Tour* (see page 15 of this workbook). Click on the down arrow next to Patient and choose Piya Jordan's room number **403**. Select **Vital Signs** as the category. Next, record the vital signs data you just collected in the last column. (*Note:* If you need help with this process, see page 16.) Now compare these findings with the data you collected earlier for this patient's vital signs. Use these earlier findings to establish a baseline for each of the vital signs.

  a. Are any of the data you collected significantly different from the baseline for a particular vital sign?

    Circle One: Yes   No

  b. If "Yes," which data are different?

■ PHYSICAL ASSESSMENT

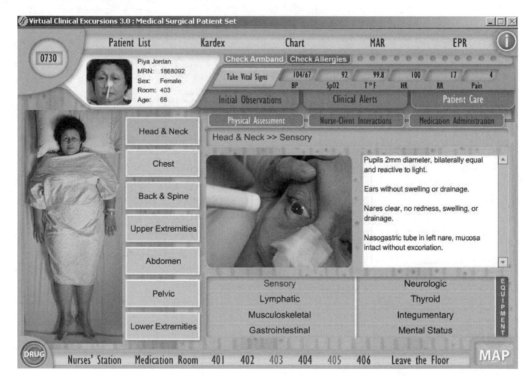

After you have finished examining the EPR for vital signs, click **Exit EPR** to return to Room 403. Click **Patient Care** and then **Physical Assessment**. Think about what information you received in report, as well as what you may have learned about this patient from the chart. What area(s) of examination should you pay most attention to at this time? Is there any equipment you should be monitoring? Conduct a physical assessment of the body areas and systems that you consider priorities for Piya Jordan. For example, select **Head & Neck**; then click on and assess **Sensory** and **Lymphatic**. Complete any other assessment(s) you think are necessary at this time. In the following table, record the data you collected during this examination.

Area of Examination	Findings
Head & Neck Sensory	
Head & Neck Lymphatic	

After you have finished collecting these data, return to the EPR. Compare the data that were already in the record with those you just collected.

    a.   Are any of the data you collected significantly different from the baselines for this patient?

        Circle One: Yes   No

    b.   If "Yes," which data are different?

■ **NURSE-CLIENT INTERACTIONS**

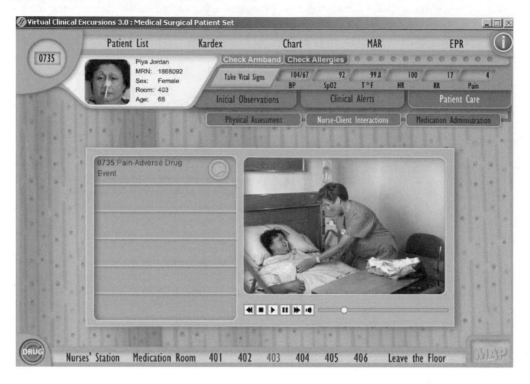

Click on **Patient Care** from inside Piya Jordan's room (403). Now click on **Nurse-Client Interactions** to access a short video titled **Pain—Adverse Drug Event**, which is available for viewing at 0735 (based on the virtual clock in the upper left corner of your screen). To begin the video, click on the arrow next to its title. You will observe a nurse communicating with Piya Jordan and her daughter. There are many variations of nursing practice, some exemplifying "best" practice and some not. Note whether the nurse in this interaction displays professional behavior and compassionate care. Are her words congruent with what is going on with the patient? Does this interaction "feel right" to you? If not, how would you handle this situation differently? Explain.

Note: If the video you wish to view is not listed, this means you have not yet reached the correct virtual time to view that video. Check the virtual clock; you may return to access the video once its designated time has occurred—as long as you do so within the corresponding period of care.

At least one Nurse-Client Interactions video is available during each period of care. Viewing these videos can help you learn more about what is occurring with a patient at a certain time and also prompt you to discriminate between nurse communications that are ideal and those that need improvement. Compassionate care and the ability to communicate clearly are essential components of delivering quality nursing care, and it is during your clinical time that you will begin to refine these skills.

■ COLLECTING AND EVALUATING DATA

Each of the activities you perform in the Patient Care environment generates a great deal of assessment data. Remember that after you collect data, you can record your findings in the EPR. You can also review the EPR, patient's chart, videos, and MAR at any time. You will get plenty of practice collecting and then evaluating data in context of the patient's course.

Now, here's an important question for you:

> Did the previous sequence of exercises provide the most efficient way to assess Piya Jordan?

For example, you went to the patient's room to get vital signs, then back to the EPR to enter data and compare your findings with extant data. Next, you went back to the patient's room to do a physical examination, then again back to the EPR to enter and review data. If this back-and-forth process of data collection and recording seemed inefficient, remember the following:

- Plan all of your nursing activities to maximize efficiency while at the same time optimizing quality of patient care. (Think about what data you might need to perform certain tasks. For example, do you need to check a heart rate before administering a cardiac medication or check an IV site before starting an infusion?)

- You collect a tremendous amount of data when you work with a patient. Very few people can accurately remember all these data for more than a few minutes. Develop efficient assessment skills, and record data as soon as possible after collecting them.

- Assessment data are only the starting point for the nursing process.

Make a clear distinction between these first exercises and how you actually provide nursing care. These initial exercises were designed to involve you actively in the use of different software components. This workbook focuses on sensible practices for implementing the nursing process in ways that ensure the highest quality care of patients.

Most important, remember that a human being changes through time, and that these changes include both the physical and psychosocial facets of a person as a living organism. Think about this for a moment. Some patients may change physically in a very short time (a patient with emerging myocardial infarction) or more slowly (a patient with a chronic illness). Patients' overall physical and psychosocial conditions may improve or deteriorate. They may have effective coping skills and familial support, or they may feel alone and full of despair. In fact, each individual is a complex mix of physical and psychosocial elements, and at least some of these elements usually change through time.

Thus it is crucial *not* to think of the nursing process as a simple one-time, five-step procedure:

- Assessment
- Nursing Diagnosis
- Planning
- Implementation
- Evaluation

Rather, the nursing process should be utilized as a creative and systematic approach to delivering nursing care. Furthermore, because all living organisms are constantly changing, we must apply the nursing process over and over. Each time we follow the nursing process for an individual patient, we refine our understanding of that patient's physical and psychosocial conditions based on collection and analysis of many different types of data. *Virtual Clinical Excursions—Medical-Surgical* will help you develop both the creativity and the systematic approach needed to become a nurse who is equipped to deliver the highest quality care to all patients.

REDUCING MEDICATION ERRORS

Earlier in this detailed tour, you learned the basic steps of medication preparation and administration. The following simulations will allow you to practice those skills further—with an increased emphasis on reducing medication errors by using the Medication Scorecard to evaluate your work.

Sign in to work at Pacific View Regional Hospital for Period of Care 1. (*Note:* If you are already working with another patient or during another period of care, click on **Leave the Floor** and then **Restart the Program**; then sign in.)

From the Patient List, select Clarence Hughes. Then click on **Go To Nurses' Station**. Complete the following steps to prepare and administer medications to Clarence Hughes.

- Click on **Medication Room**.
- Click on **MAR** to determine prn medications that have been ordered for Clarence Hughes to address his constipation and pain. (*Note:* You may click on **Review MAR** at any time to verify correct medication order. Remember to look at the patient name on the MAR to make sure you have the correct patient's record—you must click on the correct room number within the MAR.) Click on **Return to Medication Room** after reviewing the correct MAR.
- Click on **Unit Dosage** (or on the Unit Dosage cabinet); from the close-up view, click on drawer **404**.
- Select the medications you would like to administer. After each selection, click **Put Medication on Tray**. When you are finished selecting medications, click **Close Drawer**.
- Click on **View Medication Room**.
- Click on **Automated System** (or on the Automated System unit itself). Click **Login**.
- On the next screen, specify the correct patient and drawer location.
- Select the medication you would like to administer and click on **Put Medication on Tray**. Repeat this process if you wish to administer other medications from the Automated System.
- When you are finished, click **Close Drawer**. At the bottom right corner of the next screen, click on **View Medication Room**.
- From the Medication Room, click on **Preparation** (or on the preparation tray).
- From the list of medications on your tray, choose the correct medication to administer.
- Click **Next**, specify the correct patient to administer this medication to, and click **Finish**.
- Repeat the previous two steps until all medications that you want to administer are prepared.
- You can click on **Review Your Medications** and then on **Return to Medication Room** when ready. Once you are back in the Medication Room, go directly to Clarence Hughes' room by clicking on **404** at bottom of screen.
- Inside the patient's room, administer the medication, utilizing the five rights of medication administration. After you have collected the appropriate assessment data and are ready for administration, click **Patient Care** and then **Medication Administration**. Verify that the correct patient and medication(s) appear in the left-hand window. Then click the down arrow next to Select. From the drop-down menu, select **Administer** and complete the Administration Wizard by providing any information requested. When the Wizard stops asking for information, click **Administer to Patient**. Specify **Yes** when asked whether this administration should be recorded in the MAR. Finally, click **Finish**.

■ **SELF-EVALUATION**

Now let's see how you did during your earlier medication administration!

- Click on **Leave the Floor** at the bottom of your screen. From the Floor Menu, select **Look at Your Preceptor's Evaluation**. Then click on **Medication Scorecard**.

These resources will help you find out more about each patient's medications and possible sources of medication errors.

1. Start by examining Table A. These are the medications you should have given to Clarence Hughes during this period of care. If each of the medications in Table A has a √ by it, then you made no errors. Congratulations!

If there are some medications that have an X by them, then you made one or more medication errors.

Compare Tables A and B to determine which of the following types of errors you made: Wrong Dose, Wrong Route/Method/Site, or Wrong Time. Follow these steps:
   a. Find medications in Table A that were given incorrectly.
   b. Now see if those same medications are in Table B, which shows what you actually administered to Clarence Hughes.
   c. Comparing Tables A and B, match the Strength, Dose, Route/Method/Site, and Time for each medication you administered incorrectly.
   d. Then, using the form below, list the medications given incorrectly and mark the errors you made for each medication.

Medication	Strength	Dosage	Route	Method	Site	Time
	❑	❑	❑	❑	❑	❑
	❑	❑	❑	❑	❑	❑
	❑	❑	❑	❑	❑	❑
	❑	❑	❑	❑	❑	❑

2. To help you reduce future medication errors, consider the following list of possible reasons for errors.

- Did not check drug against MAR for correct patient, correct date, correct time, correct drug, and correct dose.
- Did not check drug dose against MAR three times.
- Did not open the unit dose package in the patient's room.
- Did not correctly identify the patient using two identifiers.
- Did not administer the drug on time.
- Did not verify patient allergies.
- Did not check the patient's current condition or vital sign parameters.
- Did not consider why the patient would be receiving this drug.
- Did not question why the drug was in the patient's drawer.
- Did not check the physician's order and/or check with the pharmacist when there was a question about the drug or dose.
- Did not verify that no adverse effects had occurred from a previous dose.

Based on these possibilities, determine how you made each error and record the reason into the form below:

Medication	Reason for Error

3. Look again at Table B. Are there medications listed that are not in Table A? If so, you gave a medication to Clarence Hughes that he should not have received. Complete the following exercises to help you understand how such an error might have been made.

a. Perhaps you gave a medication that was on Clarence Hughes' MAR for this period of care, without recognizing that a change had occurred in the patient's condition that should have caused you to reconsider. Review patient records as necessary and complete the following form:

Medication	Possible Reasons Not to Give This Medication

b. Another possibility is that you gave Clarence Hughes a medication that should have been given at a different time. Check his MAR and complete the form below to determine whether you made a Wrong Time error:

Medication	Given to Clarence Hughes at What Time	Should Have Been Given at What Time

c. Maybe you gave another patient's medication to Clarence Hughes. In this case, you made a Wrong Patient error. Check the MARs of other patients and use the form below to determine whether you made this type of error:

Medication	Given to Clarence Hughes	Should Have Been Given to

4. The Medication Scorecard provides some other interesting sources of information. For example, if there is a medication selected for Clarence Hughes but it was not given to him, there will be an X by that medication in Table A, but it will not appear in Table B. In that case, you might have given this medication to some other patient, which is another type of Wrong Patient error. To investigate further, look at Table D, which lists the medications you gave to other patients. See whether you can find any medications for Clarence Hughes that were given to another patient by mistake. Before making any decisions, be sure to cross-check the other patients' MAR because they may have had the same medication ordered. Use the following form to record your findings:

Medication	Should Have Been Given to Clarence Hughes	Given by Mistake to

5. Now take some time to review the exercises you just completed. Use the form below to create an overall analysis of what you have learned. Once again, record each of the medication errors you made, including the type of each error. Then, for each error you made, indicate specifically what you would do differently to prevent this type of error from occurring again.

Medication	Type of Error	Error Prevention Tactic

Submit this form to your instructor if required as a graded assignment, or simply use these exercises to improve your understanding of medication errors and how to reduce them.

Name: _____   Date: _____

The following icons are used throughout the workbook to help you quickly identify particular activities and assignments:

 Indicates a reading assignment—tells you which textbook chapter(s) you should read before starting each lesson

 Indicates a writing activity

 Marks the beginning of an interactive CD-ROM activity—signals you to open or return to your *Virtual Clinical Excursions—Medical-Surgical* CD-ROM

 Indicates additional CD-ROM instructions

 Indicates questions and activities that require you to consult your textbook

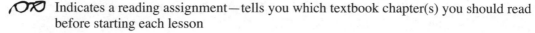 Indicates the approximate time required to complete an exercise

LESSON **1**

Health Assessment

/OO **Reading Assignment:** The Aging Population (Chapter 2)

Patients: Piya Jordan, Room 403
Clarence Hughes, Room 404
Pablo Rodriguez, Room 405

Goal: Accurately obtain a complete health assessment.

Objectives:

1. Describe appropriate guidelines for the health history interview.
2. Obtain a complete health history of an assigned patient.
3. Prioritize data collection from a patient in an acute situation.
4. Describe the four primary techniques utilized in physical examination.
5. Perform and document a thorough physical examination on an assigned patient.

In this lesson you will discuss and obtain a complete health assessment on assigned patients. Begin this activity by reviewing the general concepts presented in your textbook. Answer the following questions to solidify your understanding of culture.

Exercise 1

Clinical Preparation: Writing Activity

20 minutes

1. What environmental factors are most conducive for a health history interview?

2. Describe appropriate guidelines related to the patient when conducting a health history interview.

3. Describe appropriate guidelines related to the interviewer when conducting a health history interview.

4. Identify the five major components of the health history.

5. Document and describe the four primary techniques utilized in a physical assessment by completing the table below.

Technique	Description
a.	
b.	
c.	
d.	

Exercise 2

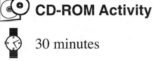 **CD-ROM Activity**

30 minutes

- Sign in to work at Pacific View Regional Hospital for Period of Care 1. (*Note:* If you are already in the virtual hospital from a previous exercise, click on **Leave the Floor** and then **Restart the Program** to get to the sign-in window.)
- From the Patient List, select Piya Jordan (Room 403) and Pablo Rodriguez (Room 405).
- Click on **Go to Nurses' Station**.
- Click on **403** to go to Piya Jordan's room.

1. As a student nurse, you are entering the patient's room to obtain a health history for your assigned clinical preparation documentation. What do you learn about Piya Jordan's state of mind from the initial observation?

2. Can you obtain an accurate history from Piya Jordan at this time? Why or why not?

3. You know that your instructor will still expect you to know Piya Jordan's current history. Other than reading the physician's H&P, how could you obtain this information?

→ • Click on **Nurses' Station**.
   • Click on **Chart** and then on **405** to obtain Pablo Rodriguez's record.
   • Click on **Nursing Admission**.

4. Health assessment begins with the health history. You will now document a health history on Pablo Rodriguez using the long format discussed in your textbook. This format differs from that used in the Pacific View Regional Hospital chart on your CD-ROM. Read the Nursing Admission form to obtain and record the information requested below and on the next four pages. If the information is not available, write N/A.

Biographic Data

Current Health
   Chief complaint

   Symptom analysis

Past Health History

Family Health History

Psychosocial History
   Psychosocial risk factors
      Social history

      Personal and family history

      Level of stress

Gastrointestinal

Genitourinary

Health Risk Appraisal

5. Compare your health history format with the one used in the chart on your CD-ROM. Which format do you believe directs the nurse to obtain the most complete health history? Explain.

Exercise 3

CD-ROM Activity

40 minutes

- Sign in to work at Pacific View Regional Hospital for Period of Care 2. (*Note:* If you are already in the virtual hospital from a previous exercise, click on **Leave the Floor** and then **Restart the Program** to get to the sign-in window.)
- From the Patient List, select Clarence Hughes (Room 404) and Pablo Rodriguez (Room 405).
- Click on **Go to Nurses' Station**.
- Click on **404** to enter Clarence Hughes' room.

1. As a student nurse, you are entering Clarence Hughes' room to obtain a health history for your assigned clinical preparation documentation. What do you learn about Clarence Hughes from the initial observation?

Usual coping pattern

Changes in neurophysiologic function

Level of understanding about health problems

Mental status

Personality style

Major psychosocial reactions

Psychologic Assessment
General appearance

Motor activity

Behavior

Mental status

Level of consciousness

Orientation to person, place, time, and circumstances

Mood and affect

Speech and communication (language)

Thought process and content

Attention span

Memory: immediate, recent, and remote

General fund of knowledge

Calculations

Abstract reasoning and thinking

Perceptual distortion

Judgment

Insight

Other Psychologic Factors
Motivation

Personal strengths

Values and beliefs

Spirituality

Sociologic Assessment
Psychosocial development

Social network

Socioeconomic status

Lifestyle

Sexuality

Cultural Asssessment

Review of Systems
Neurologic

Musculoskeletal

Cardiovascular

Respiratory

Integumentary

2. Would it be appropriate to obtain a complete history at this time? If not, how would you adapt your data collection at this point?

 • Click on **405** to enter Pablo Rodriguez's room.
• Click on **Patient Care**.

3. Health assessment continues with the physical examination. You will now perform a head-to-toe assessment on Pablo Rodriguez. For each of the main body areas listed in the table below and on the next three pages, click on the corresponding yellow button on your screen. Then select each of the assessment subcategories and record your findings in the middle column of the table. (*Note:* You will complete the table in questions 4 and 5.)

Area Assessed	Assessment Findings	Technique(s) Used
Head & Neck Sensory		
Lymphatic		
Musculoskeletal		
Gastrointestinal		
Neurologic		
Thyroid		

Area Assessed	Assessment Findings	Technique(s) Used
Integumentary		
Mental Status		
Chest Integumentary		
Cardiovascular		
Breasts		
Respiratory		
Musculoskeletal		
Back & Spine Integumentary		
Musculoskeletal		
Respiratory		
Upper Extremities Integumentary		

Area Assessed	Assessment Findings	Technique(s) Used
Musculoskeletal		
Vascular		
Neurologic		
Abdomen Integumentary		
Musculoskeletal		
Gastrointestinal		
Reproductive		
Pelvic Integumentary		
Gastrointestinal		
Urologic		
Reproductive		

Area Assessed	Assessment Findings	Technique(s) Used
Lower Extremities Integumentary		
Musculoskeletal		
Vascular		
Neurologic		

4. Identify the technique(s) of examination that would be used to obtain each of the findings you recorded in the table in question 3. Document these techniques in the last column of the table.

5. Review the physical examination data collected in question 3. Underline any abnormal assessment data.

6. Based on the abnormal data identified in question 5, summarize Pablo Rodriguez's health problems.

7. Identify two priority nursing diagnoses for Pablo Rodriguez.

LESSON 2

End-of-Life Care

Reading Assignment: Palliative and End-of-Life Care (Chapter 8)

Patient: Pablo Rodriguez, Room 405

Goal: Demonstrate understanding and appropriate application of end-of-life concepts in nursing practice.

Objectives:

1. Identify appropriate application of palliative care concepts for a patient with a terminal illness.
2. Assess for and identify common clinical manifestations present at end of life.
3. Choose interventions appropriate to relieve clinical manifestations in a terminally ill patient.
4. Describe appropriate communication techniques when dealing with a terminally ill patient and family.
5. Discuss ethical issues related to providing pain relief during end-of-life care.

In this lesson you will describe, plan, and evaluate the care of a patient with a terminal illness that is no longer responding to therapy. Pablo Rodriguez is a 71-year-old male suffering from advanced small-cell lung carcinoma diagnosed 1 year ago.

Exercise 1

Clinical Preparation: Writing Activity

15 minutes

1. What are the goals for end-of-life care?

2. Describe the diagnostic criteria for clinical diagnosis of brain death in adults as recommended by the Quality Standards Subcommittee of the American Academy of Neurology in 1995.

3. What is the defined purpose of palliative care?

4. What two criteria must be present for admission to a hospice program?

Exercise 2

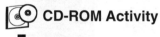 **CD-ROM Activity**

30 minutes

- Sign in to work at Pacific View Regional Hospital for Period of Care 3. (*Note:* If you are already in the virtual hospital from a previous exercise, click on **Leave the Floor** and then **Restart the Program** to get to the sign-in window.)
- From the Patient List, select Pablo Rodriguez (Room 405).
- Click on **Go to Nurses' Station**.
- Click on **Chart** and then on **405**.
- Click on the **Emergency Department** tab and review this record.

1. Why was Pablo Rodriguez admitted to the hospital?

2. What are his primary and secondary diagnoses?

 • Click on **Nursing Admission**.

3. What does the admitting nurse document as this patient's anticipated needs for support at the time of discharge?

4. Does the patient have a signed advance directive?

 5. What does the Patient Self-Determination Act of 1991 require health care agencies to provide to patients without an advance directive? (*Hint:* See textbook page 241.)

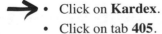 • Click on **Nurse's Notes**.

6. Based on available documentation, do you think the admitting nurse complied with the Patient Self-Determination Act of 1991?

• Click on **Kardex**.
• Click on tab **405**.

7. What is Pablo Rodriguez's code status? Is this appropriate based on the reason for this admission? (*Hint:* See your answer for question 1.) Explain.

➡ • Click on **Return to Nurses' Station**.
   • Click on **405**.
   • Select **Patient Care**.
   • Click on **Nurse-Client Interactions**.
   • Select and view the viseo titled **1530: Decision—End-of-Life Care**. (*Note:* If this video title is not available, check the virtual clock to see whether enough time has elapsed. The video cannot be viewed before its specified time.)

8. What is Pablo Rodriguez telling the nurse?

9. What therapeutic communication techniques is the nurse using? Are they effective? What other technique(s) might have been used?

 10. What would you do if Pablo Rodriguez asked you to administer a lethal dose of morphine to "stop my pain and help me die with dignity"?

➡ • Now select and view the video titled **0735: Patient Perceptions**.

10. Now that his pain has been controlled, what two physical symptoms does Pablo Rodriguez complain of? How would you intervene to relieve these discomforts?

11. Recall the goals for end-of-life care as noted in your preclinical assignment. Are these being met for Pablo Rodriguez? Explain.

11. What legal term would apply if you were to comply with this request?

Exercise 3

CD-ROM Activity

⏱ 45 minutes

- Sign in to work at Pacific View Regional Hospital for Period of Care 1. (*Note:* If you are already in the virtual hospital from a previous exercise, click on **Leave the Floor** and then **Restart the Program** to get to the sign-in window.)
- From the Patient List, select Pablo Rodriguez (Room 405).
- Click on **Go to Nurses' Station**.
- Click on **405**.

1. According to the Initial Observation report on Pablo Rodriguez, what physical symptom of distress is he displaying?

2. How would you intervene to alleviate his symptoms? Provide rationales for your interventions. (*Hint:* If you need help, go to the patient's chart to review the physician's orders. The Drug Guide in the Nurses' Station may provide rationales for medication administration.)

→ • Click on **Nurses' Station**.
   • Click on **EPR**.
   • Click **Login**.
   • Select **405** from the drop-down menu next to Patient.
   • With **Vital Signs** as the selected category, find the vital sign assessment documented at 0700. (*Hint:* Use the backward and forward arrows to scroll between times.)

3. Describe Pablo Rodriguez's pain assessment.

4. What interventions would be appropriate to relieve this pain?

Now let's check the patient's current vital signs.

→ • Click on **Exit EPR**.
   • Click on **Room 405** at the bottom of your screen.
   • Click on **Take Vital Signs**. (Note that pain assessment is now considered the fifth vital sign.)

5. Based on the EPR data and Pablo Rodriguez's current pain rating, is the morphine providing effective relief? Explain.

→ • Click on **Patient Care**.
   • From the list of body areas (the yellow buttons), click on **Abdomen**.
   • From the system subcategories, click on **Gastrointestinal**.

6. Document your assessment findings below. What is the significance of these findings? How do they relate to Pablo Rodriguez's diagnosis and/or treatment?

7. How would you intervene to prevent potential complications related to the above findings?

→ • Click on **Nurse-Client Interactions**.
   • Select and view the video titled **0730: Symptom Management**. (*Note:* If this video title is not available, check the virtual clock to see whether enough time has elapsed. The video cannot be viewed before its specified time.)

8. Describe Pablo Rodriguez's emotional distress as displayed in this video.

9. What nursing interventions would be appropriate to help this patient cope?

11. What legal term would apply if you were to comply with this request?

Exercise 3

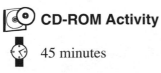 **CD-ROM Activity**

45 minutes

- Sign in to work at Pacific View Regional Hospital for Period of Care 1. (*Note:* If you are already in the virtual hospital from a previous exercise, click on **Leave the Floor** and then **Restart the Program** to get to the sign-in window.)
- From the Patient List, select Pablo Rodriguez (Room 405).
- Click on **Go to Nurses' Station**.
- Click on **405**.

1. According to the Initial Observation report on Pablo Rodriguez, what physical symptom of distress is he displaying?

2. How would you intervene to alleviate his symptoms? Provide rationales for your interventions. (*Hint:* If you need help, go to the patient's chart to review the physician's orders. The Drug Guide in the Nurses' Station may provide rationales for medication administration.)

- Click on **Nurses' Station**.
- Click on **EPR**.
- Click **Login**.
- Select **405** from the drop-down menu next to Patient.
- With **Vital Signs** as the selected category, find the vital sign assessment documented at 0700. (*Hint:* Use the backward and forward arrows to scroll between times.)

3. Describe Pablo Rodriguez's pain assessment.

4. What interventions would be appropriate to relieve this pain?

Now let's check the patient's current vital signs.

- Click on **Exit EPR**.
- Click on **Room 405** at the bottom of your screen.
- Click on **Take Vital Signs**. (Note that pain assessment is now considered the fifth vital sign.)

5. Based on the EPR data and Pablo Rodriguez's current pain rating, is the morphine providing effective relief? Explain.

- Click on **Patient Care**.
- From the list of body areas (the yellow buttons), click on **Abdomen**.
- From the system subcategories, click on **Gastrointestinal**.

6. Document your assessment findings below. What is the significance of these findings? How do they relate to Pablo Rodriguez's diagnosis and/or treatment?

7. How would you intervene to prevent potential complications related to the above findings?

 • Click on **Nurse-Client Interactions**.
 • Select and view the video titled **0730: Symptom Management**. (*Note:* If this video title is not available, check the virtual clock to see whether enough time has elapsed. The video cannot be viewed before its specified time.)

8. Describe Pablo Rodriguez's emotional distress as displayed in this video.

9. What nursing interventions would be appropriate to help this patient cope?

• Now select and view the video titled **0735: Patient Perceptions**.

10. Now that his pain has been controlled, what two physical symptoms does Pablo Rodriguez complain of? How would you intervene to relieve these discomforts?

11. Recall the goals for end-of-life care as noted in your preclinical assignment. Are these being met for Pablo Rodriguez? Explain.

LESSON **3**

Perioperative Care

/OᏇ **Reading Assignment:** Preoperative Care (Chapter 13)
Postoperative Care (Chapter 15)

Patients: Piya Jordan, Room 403
Clarence Hughes, Room 404

Goal: Utilize the nursing process to competently care for perioperative patients.

Objectives:

1. Document a complete history and physical on a preoperative patient.
2. Identify appropriate rationale for preoperative orders on an assigned patient.
3. Evaluate completeness of preoperative teaching on a patient scheduled for surgery.
4. Document a focused assessment on a patient transferred from PACU to a medical-surgical unit.
5. Plan appropriate interventions to prevent postoperative complications in an assigned patient.
6. Utilize the nursing process to correctly administer scheduled and prn medications to an assigned patient.

In this lesson you will learn the essentials of caring for patients in both the preoperative and postoperative stages of surgery. You will document assessments, plan, implement, and evaluate care given. Piya Jordan is a 68-year-old female admitted with nausea and vomiting for 3 days. Clarence Hughes is a 73-year-old male admitted for an elective knee replacement.

Exercise 1

CD-ROM Activity

⏱ 40 minutes

- Sign in to work at Pacific View Regional Hospital for Period of Care 1. (*Note:* If you are already in the virtual hospital from a previous exercise, click on **Leave the Floor** and then **Restart the Program** to get to the sign-in window.)
- From the Patient List, select Piya Jordan (Room 403).
- Click on **Go to Nurses' Station**.
- Click on **Chart** and then on **403**.
- Click on **Emergency Department**.

1. What day and time did Piya Jordan arrive in the Emergency Department?

2. What complaints (problems) brought her to the ED?

3. What were her primary and secondary admitting diagnoses?

➡ • Click on **Nursing Admission**.

4. Important areas of data collection for the health history during the preoperative period are listed below and on the next two pages. Using the Nursing Admission form as your source, record the data collected for each area. If an area was not completed, write "No data." (*Hint:* See pages 242-250 in your textbook for clarification of each section.)

Areas of Data Collection	Piya Jordan's Data
Psychosocial assessment	
Past medical history	
Cardiac history	
Prior surgical procedures	
Prior experience with anesthesia	
Family history	

Areas of Data Collection	Piya Jordan's Data
Current medications (including use of herbs and dietary supplements)	
Allergies (including sensitivity to latex products)	
Review of Systems Cardiovascular	
Respiratory	
Neurologic	
Urinary	
Gastrointestinal	
Hepatic	
Integumentary	
Musculoskeletal	
Endocrine	
Immune	

Areas of Data Collection	Piya Jordan's Data
Fluid and electrolyte	
Nutritional status	
Functional Health Patterns Health Perception	
Health Management Pattern	
Nutritional-Metabolic Pattern	
Elimination Pattern	
Activity-Exercise Pattern	
Sleep-Rest Pattern	
Cognitive-Perceptual Pattern	
Self-Perception/Self-Concept Pattern	
Role-Relationship Pattern	
Sexuality-Reproductive Pattern	
Coping-Stress Tolerance Pattern	
Value-Belief Pattern	

→ • Click on **History and Physical**.

5. In addition to data obtained from the health history, a physical examination provides necessary and important data for the preoperative assessment. For each of the areas listed below, identify in the middle column the key items to assess (excluding history and lab results) according to your textbook (pages 251-253). In the last column, document the results from the physician's assessment as noted in the H&P. If an area was not completed, write "No data."

Physical Examination Area	Key Specific Assessments from Textbook	Results for Piya Jordan
Cardiovascular		
Respiratory		
Urinary		
Neurologic		
Hepatic		
Musculoskeletal		
Nutritional Status		

➡ • Click on **Laboratory Reports**.

6. The most common preoperative lab tests are listed below. For each test, record results for Piya Jordan. If a test was not completed, write "No data."

Lab Tests	Piya Jordan's Results
CBC	
WBC	
RBC	
Hemoglobin	
Hematocrit	
Platelets	
Electrolytes	
Glucose	
Sodium	
Potassium	
Chloride	
CO_2	
Creatinine	
BUN	
Coagulation Tests	
PTT	
PT	
INR	
Urinalysis	
ABGs	
Liver Function Tests	
Bilirubin (total)	
Protein	
Albumin	
Alkaline phosphates	
ALT (SGPT)	
AST (SGOT)	

7. Are any of Piya Jordan's lab results abnormal or of concern for a patient preparing to undergo surgery? Explain.

Exercise 2

 CD-ROM Activity

30 minutes

- Sign in to work at Pacific View Regional Hospital for Period of Care 1. (*Note:* If you are already in the virtual hospital from a previous exercise, click on **Leave the Floor** and then **Restart the Program** to get to the sign-in window.)
- From the Patient List, select Piya Jordan (Room 403).
- Click on **Go to Nurses' Station**.
- Click on **Chart** and then on **403**.
- Click on the **Consents** tab.

1. For what procedure(s) has Piya Jordan given written consent?

2. Who signed the consent form as the witness?

3. Who is responsible for providing detailed information about the procedure(s) for which the patient has given consent?

4. What is the nurse's responsibility in regard to obtaining informed consent?

• Click on **Physician's Orders**.

5. Look at the orders for Tuesday 0130. What consent was ordered?

6. By when does this consent need to be obtained?

7. What is the purpose for the mineral oil enema that was ordered to be given to Piya Jordan?

8. What diet has the physician ordered preoperatively? What is the purpose for this diet order?

9. What is the rationale for giving Piya Jordan a unit of fresh frozen plasma preoperatively?

10. What is the rationale for ordering a dose of cefotetan on call to the OR? Is this a safe order to administer to Piya Jordan? Explain why or why not.

➡ • Click on **Surgical Reports**.

11. Scroll down to the Preoperative Checklist. What preoperative teaching was completed?

12. What does the word "routines" on the checklist refer to? Explain specific items that should have been taught to Piya Jordan preoperatively.

Exercise 3

CD-ROM Activity

45 minutes

- Sign in to work at Pacific View Regional Hospital for Period of Care 1. (*Note:* If you are already in the virtual hospital from a previous exercise, click on **Leave the Floor** and then **Restart the Program** to get to the sign-in window.)
- From the Patient List, select Clarence Hughes (Room 404).
- Click on **Go to Nurses' Station**.
- Click on **EPR** and then on **Login**.
- Select **404** (from the drop-down menu box next to Patient) for Clarence Hughes' records.
- Review Vital Signs, Respiratory, Neurologic, Integumentary, IV, Wounds and Drains, and any other EPR categories necessary to answer the following question.

1. On arrival to the medical-surgical nursing unit, a postoperative patient requires an immediate focused assessment. For each area specified in the left column below, document the assessment findings recorded by the nurse on Sunday at 1600 when Clarence Hughes arrived on the medical-surgical.

Focused Assessment Areas	Clarence Hughes' Assessment Findings
Airway	
Breathing	
Mental status	
Surgical incision site	
Vital signs	
Intravenous fluids	
Other tubes and/or drains	

2. How frequently did the nurse assess Clarence Hughes' vital signs after arrival on the unit? How often do you think his vital signs should have been assessed? (*Hint:* See pages 303-305 in your textbook.)

→ • Still in the EPR, select the **Intake and Output** category.

3. In the table below, record Clarence Hughes' I&O for the past 3 days at the times specified.

	Sun 1500-2300	Mon 2300-0700	Mon 0700-1500	Mon 1500-2300	Tues 2300-0700	Tues 0700-1500	Tues 1500-2300	Wed 2300-0700
Intake								
Output								

4. Which is greater—Clarence Hughes' intake or output? By how much? Is this expected?

5. What are the possible consequences if this trend in fluid balance continues?

→ • Click on **Exit EPR**.
• Click on **Chart** and then on **404**.
• Click on **Physician's Orders**.

6. Look at the physician's postoperative orders written on Sunday at 1600. What is ordered to prevent postoperative atelectasis?

7. What additional interventions can you suggest to further prevent atelectasis?

8. What is ordered to prevent DVT?

9. Scroll up to look at the orders for Monday 0715. What did the physician order at this time to prevent DVT postoperatively?

10. What additional interventions can you suggest to further prevent DVT?

11. What wound care is ordered on Sunday?

12. At what point may the dressing be removed and the incision left open to air?

→ • Click on **Return to Nurses' Station** and then on **404**.
   • Inside Clarence Hughes' room, click on **Take Vital Signs**. Review these results.
   • Next, click on **Clinical Alerts**.
   • Now select **Patient Care**.
   • Click on **Nurse-Client Interactions**.
   • Select and view the video titled **0735: Empathy**. (*Note:* If this video title is not available, check the virtual clock to see whether enough time has elapsed. The video cannot be viewed before its specified time.)

13. What is Clarence Hughes' major concern at this point?

➤ • Now click on **Medication Room**.
- From the Medication Room, click on **MAR** to determine medications that Clarence Hughes is ordered to receive at 0800 and any appropriate prn medications you may want to administer. (*Note:* You may click on **Review MAR** at any time to verify correct medication order. Remember to look at the patient name on the MAR to make sure you have the correct patient's record—you must click on the correct room number within the MAR. Click on **Return to Medication Room** after reviewing the correct MAR.)
- Click on **Unit Dosage** at the top of your screen or on the Unit Dosage cabinet to the right of Automated System.
- From the close-up view of the Unit Dosage drawers, click on drawer **404**.
- From the list of available medications in the top window, select the medication(s) you would like to administer. After each medication you select, click on **Put Medication on Tray**.
- When you have finished putting your selected medications on the tray, click on **Close Drawer**.
- Click on **View Medication Room**.
- This time, click on **Automated System** (or on the Automated System unit itself). Your name and password will automatically appear. Click on **Login**.
- In box 1, select the correct patient; in box 2, choose the appropriate Automated System Drawer for this patient. Then click on **Open Drawer**.
- From the list of available medications, select the medication(s) you would like to administer. For each one selected, click on **Put Medication on Tray**. When you are finished, click on **Close Drawer**.
- Click **View Medication Room**.
- From the Medication Room, click on **Preparation** (or on the preparation tray on the counter); then highlight the medication you want to administer. Click on **Prepare**.
- Wait for the Preparation Wizard to appear; then provide any information requested.
- Click **Next**, choose the correct patient to administer this medication to, and click **Finish**.
- Repeat the previous two steps until you have prepared all the medications you want to administer.
- You can click **Review Your Medications** and then **Return to Medication Room** when you are ready. Once you are back in the Medication Room, you may go directly to Clarence Hughes' room by clicking on **404** at bottom of screen.
- Administer the medication, utilizing the five rights of medication administration. After you have collected the appropriate assessment data and are ready for administration, click **Patient Care** and then **Medication Administration**. Verify that the correct patient and medication(s) appear in the left-hand window. Then click the down arrow next to Select. From the drop-down menu, select **Administer** and complete the Administration Wizard by providing any information requested. When the Wizard stops asking for information, click **Administer to Patient**. Specify **Yes** when asked whether this administration should be recorded in the MAR. Finally, click **Finish**.

Now let's see how you did!

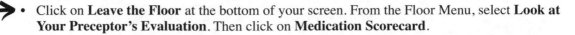 • Click on **Leave the Floor** at the bottom of your screen. From the Floor Menu, select **Look at Your Preceptor's Evaluation**. Then click on **Medication Scorecard**.

14. Note below whether or not you correctly administered the appropriate medication(s). If not, why do you think you were incorrect? According to Table C in this scorecard, what resources should be used and what important assessments should be completed before administering the medication(s)? Did you utilize these resources and perform these assessments correctly?

LESSON 4

Pain

◯◯ **Reading Assignment:** Pain (Chapter 16)

Patients: Clarence Hughes, Room 404
Pablo Rodriguez, Room 405

Goal: Demonstrate understanding and appropriate application of pain management concepts.

Objectives:

1. Define the concept of pain.
2. Describe the six dimensions of pain.
3. Describe the source and type of pain for each patient.
4. Perform a comprehensive pain assessment for each patient.
5. Identify variables that influence each patient's perception of pain.
6. Safely administer analgesic medications to a patient experiencing pain.
7. Plan appropriate nonpharmacologic measures that may be used to treat each patient's pain.

In this lesson you will evaluate the pain experience of two different patients—from assessment to management. Clarence Hughes is a 73-year-old male who is status post total knee arthroplasty. Pablo Rodriguez is a 71-year-old male admitted with advanced small-cell lung carcinoma. Begin this activity by reviewing the general concepts presented in your textbook. Answer the following questions to solidify your understanding of pain.

Exercise 1

✎ **Clinical Preparation: Writing Activity**

🕐 20 minutes

1. Using the definitions of pain provided in the textbook, describe pain in your own words.

2. Briefly describe the following six dimensions of pain discussed in your textbook.

Physiologic

Sensory

Affective

Behavioral

Cognitive

Sociocultural

Exercise 2

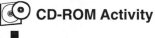 **CD-ROM Activity**

45 minutes

- Sign in to work at Pacific View Regional Hospital for Period of Care 1. (*Note:* If you are already in the virtual hospital from a previous exercise, click on **Leave the Floor** and then **Restart the Program** to get to the sign-in window.)
- From the Patient List, select Clarence Hughes (Room 404).
- Click on **Get Report**.

1. What information is obtained during report concerning Clarence Hughes' most recent pain assessment?

Now complete your own pain assessment on Clarence Hughes.

- Click on **Go to Nurses' Station**.
- Click on **404** on the bottom tool bar.
- Click on **Take Vital Signs**.

2. How does Clarence Hughes rate his pain at the present time?

- Click on **Patient Care**.

3. Perform a focused assessment on this patient. Document your findings below.

- Click on **Nurse-Client Interactions**.
- Select and view the video titled **0730: Assessment/Perception of Care**. (*Note:* If this video title is not available, check the virtual clock to see whether enough time has elapsed. The video cannot be viewed before its specified time.)

4. How does Clarence Hughes describe his pain? Describe his nonverbal communication. Do his nonverbal cues correlate with his complaint of pain?

5. The nurse asks Clarence Hughes if she may first perform an assessment prior to medicating him for pain. Is this appropriate? Why or why not?

→ • Click on **EPR** near the upper right corner of your screen.
  • Your name and password should appear automatically; click on **Login**.
  • Click on the down arrow next to the Patient field. From the drop-down menu, choose **404**.
  • Select **Vital Signs** as the category.

6. Document Clarence Hughes' pain rating and characteristics over the last 24 hours in the table provided below and on the next page. (*Note:* You will complete the table in question 7.)

→ • Click on **Exit EPR**.
  • Click on **Chart** and then on **404** for Clarence Hughes' chart.
  • Within the chart, click on the **Expired MARs** tab.

7. Review the expired MARs for Clarence Hughes, noting the times of analgesic administration. Document your findings in the far right column below and on the next page.

Time of Assessment	Pain Rating	Pain Characteristic	Name of Analgesic Administered
Tuesday 0700			
Tuesday 0815			
Tuesday 0930			
Tuesday 1230			
Tuesday 1330			

Time of Assessment	Pain Rating	Pain Characteristic	Name of Analgesic Administered
Tuesday 1500			
Tuesday 1630			
Tuesday 1700			
Tuesday 2030			
Tuesday 2300			
Wednesday 0200			
Wednesday 0715			

→ • Click on **Return to Room 404**.
• Click on **Kardex**.
• Click on **404** for Clarence Hughes' records.

8. What is the stated outcome related to comfort for Clarence Hughes? Is this a measurable outcome? How might you improve on the writing of the outcome?

9. Based on the stated outcome, review the table you completed in questions 6 and 7. Was the pain medication administered effective? Give a rationale for your answer.

10. Was the patient's pain assessed appropriately following each analgesic administration? Explain your answer.

 11. How would you classify Clarence Hughes' pain? Explain your answer. (*Hint:* See pages 339-340 of your textbook.)

12. Is the ordered analgesic medication appropriate for this type of pain? If not, what would you suggest? Are there any nonpharmacologic interventions that might be helpful for Clarence Hughes? Explain your answer.

13. What nursing assessment should be completed prior to administration of oxycodone with acetaminophen?

14. For what common side effects should the nurse monitor Clarence Hughes related to opioid use? (*Hint:* If you need help, return to the Nurses' Station and click on the **Drug Guide** on the counter.)

→ • Click on **Return to Nurses' Station** (if not already there).
   • Click on **Chart.**
   • Click on **404** for Clarence Hughes' chart.
   • Click on the **Nurse's Notes** tab and review the notes.

15. According to the note for Wednesday at 0715, which of the side effects (identified in question 14) is Clarence Hughes experiencing? What should the nurse do to treat and/or prevent this side effect?

Since Clarence Hughes received his last dose of pain medication at 0200, it is now appropriate to administer another dose. Prepare to administer a dose of analgesic to him by completing the following steps:

→ • Click on **Return to Nurses' Station**.
   • Click **Medication Room** on the bottom of your screen.
   • Access the **Automated System** by either selecting that icon at the top of screen or by clicking on the Automated System cart in center of screen.
   • Click on **Login**.
   • Choose Clarence Hughes in box 1 and Automated System Drawer (G-O) in box 2. Click **Open Drawer** and review the list of available medications. (*Note:* You may click **Review MAR** at any time to verify correct medication order. Remember to look at patient name on MAR to make sure you have the correct MAR—you must click on the correct room number within the MAR. Click on **Return to Medication Room** after reviewing the correct MAR.)
   • From the Open Drawer view, select the correct medication to administer. Click **Put Medication on Tray** and then on **Close Drawer**.
   • Click on **View Medication Room**.
   • Begin the preparation process by clicking on **Preparation** at the top of screen or clicking on the tray on the counter on the left side of the Medication Room.
   • Click **Prepare**, fill in any requested data in the Preparation Wizard, and click **Next**. Then select the correct patient and click **Finish**.
   • You can click on **Review Your Medications** and then on **Return to Medication Room** when ready. Once you are back in the Medication Room, you may go directly to Clarence Hughes' room to administer this medication by clicking on **404** at the bottom of the screen.

- Administer the medication, utilizing the five rights of medication administration. After you have collected the appropriate assessment data and are ready for administration, click **Patient Care** and then **Medication Administration**. Verify that the correct patient and medication(s) appear in the left-hand window. Then click the down arrow next to Select. From the drop-down menu, select **Administer** and complete the Administration Wizard by providing any information requested. When the Wizard stops asking for information, click **Administer to Patient**. Specify **Yes** when asked whether this administration should be recorded in the MAR. Finally, click **Finish**.

Now let's see how you did!

- Click on **Leave the Floor** at the bottom of your screen. From the Floor Menu, select **Look at Your Preceptor's Evaluation**. Then click on **Medication Scorecard**.

16. Disregard the report for the routine scheduled medications but note below whether or not you correctly administered the analgesic medication. If not, why do you think you were incorrect in administering this drug? According to Table C in this scorecard, what are the appropriate resources that should be used prior to administering this medication? Did you utilize them correctly?

Exercise 3

 CD-ROM Activity

45 minutes

- Sign in to work at Pacific View Regional Hospital for Period of Care 1. (*Note:* If you are already in the virtual hospital from a previous exercise, click on **Leave the Floor** and then **Restart the Program** to get to the sign-in window.)
- From the Patient List, select Pablo Rodriguez (Room 405).
- Click on **Get Report**.

1. What information is obtained during report concerning Pablo Rodriguez's most recent pain assessment?

Now complete your own pain assessment on this patient.

- Click on **Go to Nurses' Station**.
- Click on **405**.
- Click on **Take Vital Signs**.

2. How does Pablo Rodriguez rate his pain at the present time?

 • Click on **Patient Care**.

3. Perform a focused assessment on this patient. Document your findings below.

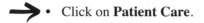 • Click on **Chart**.
  • Click on **405** for the correct patient chart.
  • Click on **Nursing Admission**.

4. Scroll down to page 22 of the Nursing Admission form. What are the aggravating and alleviating factors related to Pablo Rodriguez's pain?

5. What cultural influences are affecting this patient's perception and management of pain?

 • Click on **Return to Room 405** and then on **Patient Care**.
  • Click on **Nurse-Client Interactions**.
  • Select and view the video titled **0730: Symptom Management**. (*Note:* If this video title is not available, check the virtual clock to see whether enough time has elapsed. The video cannot be viewed before its specified time.)

➡ • Click on **EPR**.
- Click on **Login**.
- Select **405** from the drop-down menu next to Patient.
- Choose **Vital Signs** as the category.

6. In the table below, document Pablo Rodriguez's pain rating and characteristics since admission. (*Note:* You will complete the table in question 7.)

Time of Assessment	Pain Rating	Pain Characteristic	Time of Medication Administration	Name of Analgesic Administered
Tuesday 2300				
Wednesday 0300				
Wednesday 0700				

➡ • Click on **Exit EPR**.
- Click on **Chart**.
- Select **405**.
- Click on **Expired MARs**.

7. Review the expired MAR, noting the times of analgesic administration. Document your findings in the table above.

➡ • Click on **Return to Room 405**.
- Click on **Kardex**.
- Click on **405** for the correct records.

8. What is the stated outcome related to comfort for Pablo Rodriguez? Is this a measurable outcome? How might you improve on the writing of the outcome?

9. Based on the stated outcome, review the table you completed in questions 6 and 7, as well as your pain assessment in question 2. Was the pain medication administered effective? Give a rationale for your answer.

10. Was the patient's pain assessed appropriately following each analgesic administration? Explain your answer.

 11. How would you classify Pablo Rodriguez's pain? Explain your answer. (*Hint:* See page 340 of your textbook.)

12. Is the ordered analgesic medication appropriate for this type of pain? If not, what would you suggest? Are there any nonpharmacologic interventions that might be helpful for this patient? Explain your answer.

➡ • Click on **Return to Room 405**.
   • Click on **Nurse-Client Interactions**.
   • Select and view the video titled **0735: Patient Perceptions**.

13. Discuss the nurse's evaluation of Pablo Rodriguez's understanding and use of the PCA
    pump. Do you think the nurse's actions are therapeutic? If not, what other approaches
    would you suggest?

14. What nursing assessments and interventions are appropriate for patients receiving IV mor-
    phine sulfate? (*Hint:* For help, click on the **Drug** icon in the lower left corner of the screen.)

5

Fluid Imbalance

Reading Assignment: Fluid and Electrolyte Imbalance (Chapter 17)

Patients: Piya Jordan, Room 403
Patricia Newman, Room 406

Goal: Utilize the nursing process to competently care for patients with fluid imbalances.

Objectives:

1. Identify normal physiologic influences on fluid and electrolyte balance.
2. Compare and contrast causes and clinical manifestations related to water excess and water deficit.
3. Utilize laboratory data and clinical manifestations to assess fluid balance and imbalance.
4. Describe collaborative management strategies used to maintain and/or restore fluid balance.
5. Critically analyze differences in fluid balance assessment findings between two patients.
6. Develop an appropriate plan of care for patients displaying fluid imbalances.

In this lesson you will assess, plan, and implement care for two patients with similar but differing fluid imbalances. Piya Jordan is a 68-year-old female admitted with nausea and vomiting for several days following weeks of poor appetite and increasing weakness. Patricia Newman is a 61-year-old female admitted with dyspnea at rest, cough, and fever. Begin this activity by reviewing the general concepts of fluid homeostasis as presented in your textbook. Answer the following questions to cement your understanding of the normal physiologic concepts related to fluid balance.

Exercise 1

Clinical Preparation: Writing Activity

30 minutes

1. Describe the functions of body water.

2. Identify the three fluid compartments in the body and describe their composition.

3. Compare and contrast the causes and clinical manifestations of water excess (overhydration) and water deficit (dehydration) by completing the table below.

Fluid Imbalance	Causes	Clinical Manifestations
Water excess (fluid volume excess) (overhydration)		
Water deficit (fluid volume deficit) (dehydration)		

4. Match each of the following terms related to fluid volume regulation with its corresponding definition.

Term

_____ Hydrostatic pressure

_____ Colloidal oncotic pressure

_____ Diffusion

_____ Osmolarity

_____ Aldosterone

_____ Hypotonic

_____ Osmosis

_____ Antidiuretic hormone

_____ Isotonic

_____ Solute

_____ Facilitated diffusion

_____ Hypertonic

_____ Active transport

Definition

a. Movement of molecules from an area of high concentration to one of low concentration

b. Movement of water between two compartments separated by a membrane permeable to water but not to solutes; water moves from area of low solute concentration (dilute) to one of high solute concentration (concentrated)

c. The force of pressure exerted by static water in a confined space—"water-pushing" pressure

d. The concentration of solutes in 1000 mL of water

e. The solid particle dissolved in a solution

f. Any solution with a solute concentration equal to the osmolarity of normal body fluids or normal saline, about 300 mOsm/L

g. A hormone produced by the hypothalamus and released by the posterior pituitary gland to regulate body water

h. Molecules combine with a specific carrier molecule to accelerate movement from an area of high concentration to one of low concentration

i. A hormone produced by the adrenal cortex that enhances sodium retention and potassium excretion

j. Process in which molecules move against the concentration gradient; requires energy

k. Any solution with a solute concentration (osmolarity) greater than that of normal body fluids (>310 mOsm/L)

l. The osmotic pressure exerted by colloids in solution; pulls fluid from the tissue space to the vascular space

m. Any solution with a solute concentration (osmolarity) less than that of normal body fluids (<270 mOsm/L)

Exercise 2

 CD-ROM Activity

 30 minutes

- Sign in to work at Pacific View Regional Hospital for Period of Care 1. (*Note:* If you are already in the virtual hospital from a previous exercise, click on **Leave the Floor** and then **Restart the Program** to get to the sign-in window.)
- From the Patient List, select Piya Jordan (Room 403).
- Click on **Go to Nurses' Station**.
- Click on **Chart** and then on **403**.
- Click on **Emergency Department** and review this record.

1. Record findings below that support the diagnosis of dehydration (hypovolemia).

→ • Click on **Nursing Admission**.

2. Are there any additional findings noted on this document that support the diagnosis of dehydration? If so, list them below.

• Now click on the **Laboratory Reports** tab.

3. Record pertinent results below and describe the significance of each result in relation to the diagnosis of dehydration. (*Hint:* You may refer to your laboratory/diagnostic reference manual.)

4. Is Piya Jordans's fluid imbalance related to a water loss or a sodium gain?

• Click on **History and Physical**.

5. What contributing factor(s) led to this dehydration?

• Now click on **Physician's Orders** and read the initial orders for Piya Jordan.

6. Identify orders that are appropriate management strategies for the treatment of dehydration and write your findings below.

7. Develop an appropriate plan of care for Piya Jordan related to management of her fluid volume deficit.

Collaborative Plan of Care	Dehydration
Patient outcomes	
Assessment parameters	
Collaborative care interventions	

Exercise 3

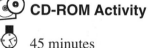 **CD-ROM Activity**

45 minutes

Now you will answer similar questions related to fluid balance for another patient and compare the findings.

- Sign in to work at Pacific View Regional Hospital for Period of Care 1. (*Note:* If you are already in the virtual hospital from a previous exercise, click on **Leave the Floor** and then **Restart the Program** to get to the sign-in window.)
- From the Patient List, select Patricia Newman (Room 406).
- Click on **Go to Nurses' Station**.
- Click on **Chart** and and then on **406**.
- Read the **Emergency Department** record.

1. Identify assessment findings related to fluid balance and record below. How do these findings differ from those for Piya Jordan? Are there any similarities?

• Click on **Nursing Admission**.

2. Are there any additional findings noted on this document related to fluid balance and/or imbalance? If so, list them below. How do they compare with findings for Piya Jordan?

 • Now review the **Laboratory Results**.

3. Record pertinent results below and describe the significance of each result in relation to fluid balance. Describe any differences between these findings and those for Piya Jordan.

4. Based on your findings, does Patricia Newman have a fluid imbalance? If so, what type?

5. What are the contributing factors for this patient's potential or actual fluid imbalance?

• Read Patricia Newman's **History and Physical**.

6. What coexisting illness might have an impact on the selection and rate of IV fluid therapy?

7. Develop an appropriate plan of care for patients with fluid volume excess by completing the chart below.

Collaborative Plan of Care	Overhydration
Patient outcomes	
Assessment parameters	
Collaborative care interventions	

LESSON 6

Electrolyte Imbalances, Part 1

Reading Assignment: Fluid and Electrolyte Imbalance (Chapter 17)

Patients: Piya Jordan, Room 403
Patricia Newman, Room 406

Goal: Utilize the nursing process to competently care for patients with electrolyte imbalances.

Objectives:

1. Describe normal physiologic influences on electrolyte balance.
2. Identify specific etiologic factors related to hypokalemia for assigned patients.
3. Research potential drug interactions related to hypokalemia for assigned patients.
4. Assess patients for clinical manifestations related to hypo- and hyperkalemia.
5. Utilize the nursing process to correctly administer IV potassium chloride per physician orders.

In this lesson you will assess, plan, and implement care for two patients with hypokalemia. Piya Jordan is a 68-year-old female admitted with nausea and vomiting for several days following weeks of poor appetite and increasing weakness. Patricia Newman is a 61-year-old female admitted with pneumonia and a history of emphysema for 12 years. Begin this activity by reviewing the general functions of electrolytes within the body as presented in your textbook. Answer the following questions to cement your understanding of the normal physiologic concepts related to potassium balance.

Exercise 1

Clinical Preparation: Writing Activity

20 minutes

1. Define the following terms.

    a. Ion

97

Copyright © 2007 by Mosby, Inc., an affiliate of Elsevier Inc. All rights reserved.

b. Cation

c. Anion

d. Valence

2. Identify the following electrolytes.

a. Primary ICF cation

b. Primary ICF anion

c. Primary ECF cation

d. Primary ECF anion

3. Identify the functions of potassium within the body.

4. Describe the physiologic influences on potassium balance.

5. Identify potential causes of hypokalemia.

6. Identify potential causes of hyperkalemia.

Exercise 2

 CD-ROM Activity

45 minutes

- Sign in to work at Pacific View Regional Hospital for Period of Care 1. (*Note:* If you are already in the virtual hospital from a previous exercise, click on **Leave the Floor** and then **Restart the Program** to get to the sign-in window.)
- From the Patient List, select Piya Jordan (Room 403).
- Click on **Go to Nurses' Station**.
- Click on **Chart** and then on **403**.
- Click on **Laboratory Reports**.

1. What was Piya Jordan's initial potassium level on Monday at 2200?

→ • Click on **Emergency Department** and review this record.

2. What would be the most likely cause for hypokalemia in this patient?

3. What did the physician order to treat this electrolyte imbalance? Is this appropriate? Are the dilution and rate safe to administer?

 • Click again on **Laboratory Reports**.

4. What was Piya Jordan's potassium level for Tuesday at 0630? Was the physician's order for potassium effective? Is there any cause for concern?

 • Click on **Return to Nurses' Station**.
   • Click on **403** to go to the patient's room.
   • Click on **Patient Care**.

5. Complete a physical assessment on Piya Jordan, specifically looking for clinical manifestations of hypokalemia. (*Hint:* Refer to your textbook on pages 374-377.) Document your findings in the chart below and underline or highlight those that correlate with hypokalemia.

Areas Assessed	Findings on Physical Examination
Cardiovascular	
Respiratory	

Areas Assessed	Findings on Physical Examination
Neuromuscular	
Gastrointestinal	
Renal	

6. Explain the underlying pathophysiology of the assessment findings you recorded in question 5 related to hypokalemia.

7. What is the potassium level that was drawn on Wednesday at 0630?

8. Explain the etiology for this recurrence of hypokalemia.

 • Click on **Chart** and then on **403**.
   • Click on **Physician's Orders**.

9. What did the physician order in response to today's potassium level?

Prepare to administer this ordered dose of potassium chloride to Piya Jordan by completing the following steps.

• Click on **Return to Room 403**.
   • Click **Medication Room** on the bottom of your screen.

- Click on **IV Storage** near the top of your screen (*Note:* You can also click on any of the three bins just above the refrigerator.) Either of these methods will bring up a close-up view of the IV storage bins.

- Click on the bin labeled **Small Volume** and review the list of available medications. (*Note:* You may click on **Review MAR** at any time to verify correct medication order. Remember to look at the patient name on the MAR to make sure you have the correct patient's record— you must click on the correct room number within the MAR. Click on **Return to Medication Room** after reviewing the correct MAR.)

- From the list of medications in the bin, select **potassium chloride**. Then click **Put Medication on Tray** and **Close Bin**.

- Click **View Medication Room**.

- Click on **Preparation** at the top of the screen or on the preparation tray on the counter. Select the correct medication to administer; then click **Prepare**.

- Wait for instructions or questions from the Preparation Wizard. Then click **Next**.

- Choose the correct patient to administer this medication to. Click **Finish**.

- You can click **Review Your Medications** and then **Return to Medication Room** when ready. From the Medication Room, go directly to Piya Jordan's room by clicking on **403** at bottom of screen.

Prior to administering intravenous medications, the patient's IV site must first be assessed.

- Click on **Patient Care**.
- Click on **Upper Extremities**.
- Select **Integumentary** from the system subcategories.

10. Document the IV site assessment findings below. Is it appropriate to administer the IV potassium at this time? What other steps should you take to ensure you have adequately addressed the five rights of medication administration?

- After you have collected the appropriate assessment data and are ready for administration, click on **Medication Administration**. (*Note:* If you are not still in the Patient Care screen, you will need to first click **Patient Care** and then choose **Medication Administration**.)

- To the right of the medication name, next to Select, click the down arrow and choose **Administer** from the drop-down menu.

- Complete the Administration Wizard and click **Administer to Patient** when done.

- Check **Yes** when asked whether this drug administration should be documented on the MAR.

- Now click on **MAR** at the top of your screen.

11. What are Piya Jordan's scheduled AM medications?

12. What assessment factors should the nurse consider before administering digoxin to Piya Jordan?

13. Following data collection on the identified assessment areas in question 12, what nursing intervention(s) would be most appropriate? Explain.

14. Piya Jordan complains of pain at the IV site while the potassium is infusing. What interventions might be used at this point?

Now let's see how you did!

 • Click on **Leave the Floor at** the bottom of your screen. From the Floor Menu, select **Look at Your Preceptor's Evaluation**. Then click on **Medication Scorecard**.

15. Disregard the report for the routine scheduled medications, but note below whether or not you correctly administered the potassium chloride. If not, why do you think you were incorrect in administering this drug? According to Table C in this scorecard, what are the appropriate resources that should be used and important assessments that should be completed prior to administering this medication? Did you utilize and perform them correctly?

Exercise 3

 CD-ROM Activity

 30 minutes

- Sign in to work at Pacific View Regional Hospital for Period of Care 1. (*Note:* If you are already in the virtual hospital from a previous exercise, click on **Leave the Floor** and then **Restart the Program** to get to the sign-in window.)
- Assign yourself to care for Patricia Newman (Room 406).
- Click on **Go to Nurses' Station**.
- Click on **Chart** and then on **406**.
- Click on **Laboratory Reports**.

1. What was Patricia Newman's initial potassium level this morning?

➡ • Click on **History and Physical**.

2. What would be the most likely cause for hypokalemia in this patient?

➡ • Click on **Physician's Orders**.

3. What did the physician order to treat this electrolyte imbalance?

• Click on **Return to Nurses' Station**.
   • Click on **MAR** and then on **406**.

   4. What is missing from this order?

   5. Where could you verify this missing information?

   6. What is the difference between the treatment of hypokalemia for Piya Jordan and that for Patricia Newman? Provide a rationale for the difference.

 • Click on **Return to Nurses' Station**.
   • Click on **Chart** and then on **406**.
   • Click on **Physician's Orders**.

   7. Look again at the physician's orders. Is there an order for any follow-up lab work?

   8. What is the nurse's responsibility in regard to follow-up lab work? How would you handle this situation?

→ • Click on **Return to Nurses' Station**.
- Click on **406** to go to Patricia Newman's room.
- Select **Patient Care**.
- Click on **Nurse-Client Interactions**.
- Select and view the video titled **0740: Evaluation—Response to Care**. (*Note:* If this video title is not available, check the virtual clock to see whether enough time has elapsed. The video cannot be viewed before its specified time.)

9. Although Patricia Newman is happy that her chest does not hurt like it did, what does she verbalize as a concern?

10. What is the nurse's response to the patient's expressed concern?

11. When evaluating the care of Patricia Newman, for what potential complications of IV potassium therapy would you monitor? (*Hint:* Consult the Drug Guide by clicking on the **Drug** icon in the lower left corner of your screen.)

4. Find Pablo Rodriguez's sodium level for Wednesday at 0730. Was the physician's ordered treatment effective? Can you anticipate or suggest any changes in orders?

5. Hyponatremia can be associated with both hypovolemia (actual sodium loss) and hypervolumia (dilutional). Initially, in the ED, what do you think Pablo Rodriguez's volume status was? Explain.

→ • Click on **Return to Nurses' Station**.
   • Click on **EPR** and then on **Login**.
   • Select **405** as the patient's room and **I&O** as the category.

6. Record the I&O shift totals for Pablo Rodriguez below.

Shift Totals	Tuesday 0705	Tuesday 1505	Tuesday 2305	Wednesday 0705
Intake				
Output				

7. Based on the above I&O totals obtained after the patient received IV replacement therapy, what factor(s) may be contributing to the persistant hyponatremia? Explain.

LESSON **7**

Electrolyte Imbalances, Part 2—Gastrointestinal

Reading Assignment: Fluid and Electrolyte Imbalance (Chapter 17)

Patient: Pablo Rodriguez, Room 405

Goal: Utilize the nursing process to competently care for patients with electrolyte imbalances.

Objectives:

1. Describe the pathophysiologic basis of electrolyte imbalances noted on a specific patient.
2. Identify specific etiologic factor(s) related to hypercalcemia, hyponatremia, and hypophosphatemia in the assigned patient.
3. Assess the assigned patient for clinical manifestations related to sodium, calcium, and phosphorus imbalances.
4. Describe nursing interventions appropriate when caring for a patient with hypercalcemia, hyponatremia, and hypophosphatemia.
5. Evaluate the effectiveness of medication prescribed to treat electrolyte imbalances.

In this lesson you will assess, plan, and implement care for a patient with several electrolyte imbalances. Pablo Rodriguez is a 71-year-old male who is admitted with nausea and vomiting for several days. He has a 1-year history of lung carcinoma. Begin this activity by reviewing the general functions of specific electrolytes within the body as presented in your textbook. Answer the following questions to cement your understanding of the normal physiologic concepts related to phosphorous, sodium, chloride, and calcium balance.

Exercise 1

Clinical Preparation: Writing Activity

15 minutes

1. Prior to caring for a patient with multiple electrolyte imbalances, it is imperative that you first review and reinforce general concepts related to specific electrolytes. Using the textbook, complete the table below by providing information related to calcium, phosphorous, and sodium. Refer to this table as you proceed through the CD-ROM activity to relate textbook knowledge to actual patient care.

Electrolyte	Normal Level	Functions	Major Location (i.e., ICF or ECF)	Pathophysiologic Influences
Calcium				
Phosphorus				
Sodium				

Exercise 2

CD-ROM Activity

45 minutes

- Sign in to work at Pacific View Regional Hospital for Period of Care 1. (*Note:* If you are already in the virtual hospital from a previous exercise, click on **Leave the Floor** and then **Restart the Program** to get to the sign-in window.)
- From the Patient List, select Pablo Rodriguez (Room 405).
- Click on **Go to Nurses' Station**.
- Click on **Chart** and then on **405**.
- Click on **Laboratory Reports**.

1. Complete the table below by recording Pablo Rodriguez's serum chemistry results. Identify abnormal values by marking as H (for high) or L (for low).

Lab Test	Lab Result Tuesday 2000	Lab Result Wednesday 0730
Sodium		
Potassium		
Chloride		
Calcium		
Phosphorus		
Magnesium		

→ • Click on **Emergency Department** and review this record.

2. What would be the most likely cause for the hyponatremia noted on admission in this patient?

3. What did the physician order to treat this electrolyte imbalance?

→ • Click on **Return to Nurses' Station**.
- Click on **405**.
- Select **Patient Care**.

8. Complete a physical assessment on Pablo Rodriguez, specifically looking for clinical manifestations of hyponatremia. (*Hint:* Refer to textbook pages 371-374.) Document your findings in the table below; underline or highlight those that correlate with hyponatremia.

Areas Assessed	Findings on Physical Examination
Cardiovascular	
Respiratory	
Neuromuscular	
Gastrointestinal	

→ • Click on **Chart** and then on **405**.
   • Click on the **Nursing Admission** tab.

9. What other factors could be causing or contributing to the manifestations that you underlined or highlighted in the table in question 8?

10. Based on your answers to questions 8 and 9, what conclusion can you make regarding these clinical manifestations and Pablo Rodriguez's sodium levels?

 11. What additional clinical manifestations of hyponatremia might you expect to find in other patients with this electrolyte imbalance? (*Hint:* See textbook page 372.)

12. If Pablo Rodriguez had a sodium level of 120 (severe hyponatremia), how would the treatment vary?

Exercise 3

 CD-ROM Activity

60 minutes

- Sign in to work at Pacific View Regional Hospital for Period of Care 3. (*Note:* If you are already in the virtual hospital from a previous exercise, click on **Leave the Floor** and then **Restart the Program** to get to the sign-in window.)
- From the Patient List, select Pablo Rodriguez.
- Click on **Go to Nurses' Station**.
- Click on **Chart** and then on **405**.
- Click on the **History and Physical** tab.

1. What electrolyte imbalances did Pablo Rodriguez present with on admission?

→ • Click on **Laboratory Reports**.

2. What was Pablo Rodriguez's calcium level on admission to the ED on Tuesday evening?

3. How does this level correlate with the physician's diagnosis? Speculate as to the reason for the discrepancy.

4. What was Pablo Rodriguez's phosphorous level during the same time frame?

5. How does this relate to his calcium level? Explain the pathophysiologic rationale supporting your answer.

6. What other laboratory test(s) would give the nurse a more accurate picture of Pablo Rodriguez's calcium balance? Explain your answer.

 • Click on **History and Physical**.

7. What would be the most likely cause for hypercalcemia in this patient? (*Hint:* See pages 380-381 in your textbook.)

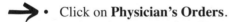 • Click on **Physician's Orders**.

8. What medication did the ED physician order to treat the hypercalcemia?

9. Describe the mechanism of action of the above medication.

10. Plicamycin can also be used to treat hypercalcemia. Why did the physician choose pamidronate over plicamycin?

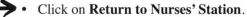 • Click on **Return to Nurses' Station**.
   • Click on the **Drug Guide** on the counter.

11. What nursing assessments are appropriate related to the administration of pamidronate?

 • Click on **Return to Nurses' Station**.
   • Click on **Chart** and then on **405**.
   • Click on **Laboratory Reports**.

12. What were Pablo Rodriguez's calcium and phosphorous levels this morning (Wednesday at 0730)?

13. Was the prescribed medication effective? Is the patient out of danger?

 • Click on **Return to Nurses' Station**.
   • Click on **Kardex** and then on tab **405**

14. What intravenous fluids is Pablo Rodriguez receiving?

15. What is the purpose of IV hydration in relation to serum calcium levels?

16. Is this the solution you would normally expect to administer to a patient with hypercalcemia? If not, what solution would you expect?

 • Click on **Return to Nurses' Station**.
   • Click on **MAR** and then on tab **405**.

17. What medication is scheduled to be administered at 1500?

18. What electrolyte imbalance will this medication correct? Explain your answer. (*Hint:* For help, consult the Drug Guide.)

19. What nursing assessments must be completed before this drug is administered?

20. Do you have any concerns regarding administering this drug at this specific time? (*Hint:* Check the patient's GI history on admission.)

 • Click on **Return to Nurses' Station**.
   • Click on **405** to go to the patient's room.
   • Click on **Patient Care**.

21. Complete a physical assessment on Pablo Rodriguez (including vital signs.) Document your findings below.

Areas Assessed	Findings on Physical Examination
Cardiovascular	
Respiratory	
Neuromuscular	
Gastrointestinal	

22. Is Pablo Rodriguez demonstrating any clinical manifestations of hypercalcemia? If yes, describe the pathophysiologic basis for the symptoms. If not, explain why not.

 23. If Pablo Rodriguez had a calcium level of 12.5, what other clinical manifestations might the nurse expect to find? (*Hint:* See pages 380-382 in your textbook.)

24. When evaluating this patient's renal output, what potential complication of hypercalcemia would you be alert for?

25. After successful treatment of Pablo Rodriguez, the nurse must be alert for overcorrecting of the electrolyte imbalance. For what clinical manifestations should the nurse monitor this patient related to hypocalcemia and hyperphosphatemia?

Acid-Base Imbalance

/OᔿO **Reading Assignment:** Acid-Base Imbalance (Chapter 18)

Patients: Jacquline Catanazaro, Room 402
Patricia Newman, Room 406

Goal: Utilize the nursing process to competently care for patients with acid-base imbalances.

Objectives:

1. Describe the pathophysiologic basis of acid-base imbalance noted in assigned patients.
2. Identify specific etiologic factor(s) related to respiratory acidosis in the assigned patients.
3. Assess the assigned patients for clinical manifestations related to respiratory acidosis.
4. Describe nursing interventions appropriate when caring for specific patients with respiratory acidosis.
5. Evaluate the effectiveness of medication prescribed to treat acid-base imbalances.

In this lesson you will assess, plan, and implement care for patients with acid-base imbalance. Jacquline Catanazaro is a 45-year-old female admitted with excerabation of asthma and schizophrenia. Patricia Newman is a 61-year-old female admitted with pneumonia and a history of emphysema for 12 years. Begin this lesson by reviewing the general concepts of acid-base balance as presented in your textbook.

Exercise 1

✎ **Clinical Preparation: Writing Activity**

⌚ 20 minutes

1. Define the following terms.

   a. Acid

b. Base

c. pH

2. Describe three methods of acid-base homeostasis by completing the following table.

	Type of Defense	Mechanisms of Action
First Line of Defense: Reacts immediately		
Second Line of Defense: Reacts within minutes		
Third Line of Defense: Reacts in 2-3 days		

Exercise 2

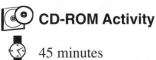 **CD-ROM Activity**

45 minutes

- Sign in to work at Pacific View Regional Hospital for Period of Care 1. (*Note:* If you are already in the virtual hospital from a previous exercise, click on **Leave the Floor** and then **Restart the Program** to get to the sign-in window.)
- From the Patient List, select Jacquline Catanazaro (Room 402).
- Click on **Go to Nurses' Station**.
- Click on **Chart** and then on **402**.
- Click on **History and Physical**.

1. Is there anything in Jacquline Catanazaro's history that would put her at risk for an acid-base imbalance?

 • Click on **Return to Nurses' Station**.
• Click on **402** to go to the patient's room.
• Select **Patient Care**.
• Click on **Nurse-Client Interactions**.
• Select and view the video titled **0730: Intervention—Airway**. (*Note:* If this video title is not available, check the virtual clock to see whether enough time has elapsed. The video cannot be viewed before its specified time.)

2. Based on Jacquline Catanazaro's history, what would you expect to be causing her respiratory distress?

3. Why is the nurse waiting until after the ABGs are being drawn to give the patient a nebulizer treatment?

• Click on **Chart** and then on **402**.
• Click on **Laboratory Reports**.

4. What are the results of Jacquline Catanazaro's two most recent ABGs? Record these below.

Results	Monday 1030	Wednesday 0730
pH		
PaO_2		
$PaCO_2$		
O_2 sat		
Bicarb		

5. How would you interpret the results in question 4? Is the acid-base imbalance compensated or uncompensated (fully or partially)? Explain your answer.

6. Since this patient's respiratory difficulties are of an acute nature, what acid-base regulation mechanisms would you expect to be working to compensate for her respiratory acidosis?

7. Based on Jacquline Catanazaro's medical diagnosis, what is the underlying pathophysiological problem leading to the respiratory acidosis?

➡ • Click on **Return to Room 402**.
• Click on **Patient Care**.

8. Do a complete physical assessment on the patient and record your findings below and on the next page.

Areas Assessed	Findings on Physical Examination
Neurologic	

Areas Assessed	Findings on Physical Examination
Musculoskeletal	
Cardiovascular	
Respiratory	
Integumentary	

9. Does this patient have any clinical manifestations of respiratory acidosis? Is so, please describe. If not, how do you explain?

→ Click on **Take Vital Signs**.

10. What is Jacquline Catanazaro's respiratory rate? How does this correlate with her respiratory acidosis?

➤ • Click on **Laboratory Reports**.

2. What are the results of Patricia Newman's two most recent ABGs? Document your findings below.

Results	Tuesday 2300	Wednesday 0500
pH		
PaO$_2$		
PaCO$_2$		
O$_2$ sat		
Bicarb		

3. How would you interpret the above results? Is the acid-base imbalance compensated or uncompensated (fully or partially)? Explain your answer.

4. Based on the chronic aspect of Patricia Newman's respiratory difficulties, what compensatory mechanisms would you expect to be working to correct the respiratory acidosis?

5. Based on the ABG results, has her condition improved or worsened since admission the evening before?

• Click on **Return to Nurses' Station**.
• Click on **Chart** and then on **406**.
• Click on **Nurse's Notes**.

6. Read the notes for Wednesday 0730. Describe the actions taken by the nurse. Are they appropriate or not? Explain you answer.

7. What additional actions do you think would be appropriate at this time?

 • Click on **Laboratory Reports**.
8. What is the patient's serum potassium level?

9. Hyperkalemia is frequently associated with acidosis as potassium moves out of the cell to compensate for hydrogen moving into the cell. How, then, would you explain the patient's hypokalemia in concert with respiratory acidosis? (*Hint:* Check the concurrent medications.)

10. Based on Patricia Newman's medical diagnosis, what is the underlying pathophysiologic problem leading to her respiratory acidosis. (*Hint:* Refer to Chapters 26 and 27 of your textbook.) How does this differ from Jacquline Catanazaro's problem in Exercise 2?

➜ • Click on **Return to Nurses' Station** and then on **406**.
   • Click on **Patient Care**.

11. Do a complete physical assessment, including vital signs, on Patricia Newman. Document your findings below.

Areas Assessed	Findings on Physical Examination
Neurologic	
Musculoskeletal	
Cardiovascular	
Respiratory	
Integumentary	

12. Does Patricia Newman have any clinical manifestations of respiratory acidosis? If so, please describe. If not, explain why not.

 13. What nursing interventions could you, as a graduate nurse, plan and implement to improve Patricia Newman's acid-base balance and prevent complications? (*Hint:* Again refer to text-book Chapters 26 and 27 for disease-specific interventions.)

LESSON 9

Cancer

Reading Assignment: Cancer (Chapter 23)
Lower Airway Problems (Chapter 26)
Hematologic Problems (Chapter 33)

Patient: Pablo Rodriguez, Room 405

Goal: Utilize the nursing process to competently care for patients with cancer.

Objectives:

1. Describe clinical manifestations and treatment for a patient with cancer.
2. Recognize special needs of patients undergoing treatment for cancer.
3. Appropriately treat a patient's symptoms related to disease process and/or side effects of treatment.
4. Discuss medications prescribed for a patient, including both expected therapeutic effects and adverse/side effects.
5. Plan appropriate general interventions to prevent and/or treat complications related to chemotherapy.

In this lesson you will learn the essentials of caring for a patient diagnosed with cancer. You will collect data, assess, plan, implement, and evaluate care given. Pablo Rodriguez is a 71-year-old male admitted with advanced small-cell lung carcinoma. Begin this lesson by reviewing the general concepts of cancer as presented in your textbook.

Exercise 1

Clinical Preparation: Writing Activity

20 minutes

1. Define the following terms.

    a. Carcinogen

    b. Oncogene

    c. Nadir

2. Briefly describe the stages of cancer development noted below and on the next page.

    a. Initiation

    b. Promotion

c. Latent period

d. Progression

3. What are the three types of therapies used to treat cancer? Describe their respective mechanisms of action.

4. What are some common side effects associated with radiation and chemotherapy?

5. Identify the common sites of distant metastasis for lung cancer.

6. List the clinical manifestations associated with lung cancer.

Exercise 2

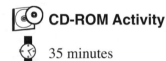 **CD-ROM Activity**

35 minutes

- Sign in to work at Pacific View Regional Hospital for Period of Care 1. (*Note:* If you are already in the virtual hospital from a previous exercise, click on **Leave the Floor** and then **Restart the Program** to get to the sign-in window.)
- From the Patient List, select Pablo Rodriguez (Room 405).
- Click on **Go to Nurses' Station**.
- Click on **Chart** and then on **405**.
- Click on **History and Physical**.

1. What is Pablo Rodriguez's main diagnosis?

2. How long ago was he diagnosed?

3. What risk factor for lung cancer is documented on the H&P?

4. What clinical manifestations documented in the physician's review of systems are related to this disease process?

5. What treatment has Pablo Rodriguez received so far?

6. How long ago did he receive his last chemotherapy?

7. What are the mechanism of action and the major side effects of doxecetaxal? (*Hint:* For help, return to the Nurses' Station and click on the **Drug Guide** on the counter.)

8. What is the nadir of docetazel? Would the patient still be having side effects from this drug? Why or why not?

→ • Click on **Physician's Notes** in the chart.

9. Look at the notes for Tuesday 1800. What type of cancer is noted? Is this the same as or different from non-small-cell cancer noted in the H&P?

Exercise 3

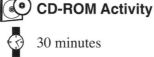 CD-ROM Activity

 30 minutes

• Sign in to work at Pacific View Regional Hospital for Period of Care 1. (*Note:* If you are already in the virtual hospital from a previous exercise, click on **Leave the Floor** and then **Restart the Program** to get to the sign-in window.)
• From the Patient List, select Pablo Rodriguez (Room 405).
• Click on **Get Report** and read the change-of-shift report.

1. What unresolved problem for Pablo Rodriguez is noted in the report?

→ • Click on **Go to Nurses' Station**.
• Click on **Chart** and then on **405**.
• Click on **Nurse's Notes**.

2. Look at the note for Wednesday at 0415. How did the nurse respond to Pablo Rodriguez's complaints? Were the nurse's actions appropriate?

3. How might you have responded differently?

→ • Click on **Return to Nurses' Station**.
  • Go to the patient's room by clicking on **405**.
  • Click on **Patient Care**.
  • Click on **Nurse-Client Interactions**.
  • Select and view the video titled **0735: Patient Perceptions**. (*Note:* If this video title is not available, check the virtual clock to see whether enough time has elapsed. The video cannot be viewed before its specified time.)

4. What are Pablo Rodriguez's two major concerns at this point?

5. What other assessment should you do before treating the patient's complaint of nausea?

→ • Click on **MAR**; then select **405** to access Pable Rodriguez's record.

6. What medications are ordered to manage the patient's pain and nausea?

7. What might the nurse question regarding these medication orders?

• Click on **Return to Room 405**.
- Click on **Chart**.
- Click on **405** for the correct chart.
- Click on **Nursing Admission**.

8. What is the patient's weight? What is this in kilograms?

 • Click on **Return to Room 405**.
- Click on the **Drug** icon in the lower left corner of the screen.

9. Calculate the maximum 24-hour dose for patients receiving this drug for nausea related to chemotherapy.

10. Calculate the maximum 24-hour dose of this drug for management of postoperative nausea and vomiting.

11. Calculate the maximum amount of metoclopramide Pablo Rodriguez could receive per 24 hours as ordered. Is it within the dosage guidelines? Is there any reason to be concerned about this dosage schedule over long periods of time?

12. What are the possible ramifications of giving high doses of this drug?

13. What are the ramifications of *not* giving metoclopramide for this patient's nausea?

14. If the nurse administers the prn Reglan at 0730, what should be done with the regularly scheduled 0800 dose?

Exercise 4

CD-ROM Activity

40 minutes

- Sign in to work at Pacific View Regional Hospital for Period of Care 2. (*Note:* If you are already in the virtual hospital from a previous exercise, click on **Leave the Floor** and then **Restart the Program** to get to the sign-in window.)
- From the Patient List, select Pablo Rodriguez (Room 405).
- Click on **Go to Nurses' Station**.
- Click on **Chart** and then on **405**.
- Click on **Laboratory Reports**.

1. Below, record Pablo Rodriguez's alkaline phosphatase and calcium levels obtained on Tuesday at 2000.

2. How do these abnormal results relate to the patient's diagnosis of cancer? (*Hint:* You may need to refer to a laboratory diagnostic reference guide.)

• Click on **Emergency Department**.

3. What is Pablo Rodriguez's chief complaint on admission to the ED? How is this related to his cancer? (*Hint:* Read the ED physician's progress notes for Tuesday at 1800.)

 • Click on **Return to Nurses' Station**.
• Click on **MAR** and then on **405**.

4. What medications still need to be given to this patient during the day shift (up to 1500)?

 • Click on the **Drug** icon in the lower left corner of the screen.
• Use the Drug Guide to answer the next three questions.

5. How does ondansetron differ from metoclopramide in regard to antiemetic mechanism of action?

6. How fast would you infuse the IV ondansetron?

7. What is the expected benefit that Pablo Rodriguez will receive from dexamethasone? Over what time period should it be administered?

• Click on **Return to Nurses' Station**.
- Click on **Chart** and then on **405**.
- Click on **Patient Education**.

8. Has any teaching yet been completed? In your opinion, what is a priority and thus should have been completed on admission?

 • Click on **Return to Nurses' Station**.
- Go to Pablo Rodriguez's room by clicking on **405**.
- Click on **Patient Care**.
- Click on **Nurse-Client Interactions**.
- Select and view the video titled **1150: Assessment—Pain**. (*Note:* If this video title is not available, check the virtual clock to see whether enough time has elapsed. The video cannot be viewed before its specified time.)

9. Why is the patient not eating?

10. Is this a normal side effect of chemotherapy?

11. How would you treat this?

➡ • Click on **Kardex** and read the outcomes.

12. What additional outcome(s) might you include for this patient?

13. What is the patient's code status? How do you feel about this in relation to patient's diagnosis and condition? What is the nurse's professional responsibility related to the patient's code status?

LESSON 10

Emphysema and Pneumonia

/O⌒Ø **Reading Assignment:** Lower Airway Problems (Chapter 26)
Chronic Respiratory Problems (Chapter 27)

Patient: Patricia Newman, Room 406

Goal: Utilize the nursing process to competently care for patients with altered oxygenation states.

Objectives:

1. Relate physical assessment findings with pathophysiologic changes of the lower respiratory tract.
2. Prioritize nursing care for a patient with altered oxygenation.
3. Evaluate laboratory results relative to the diagnosis of pneumonia and emphysema.
4. Describe pharmacologic interventions related to altered oxygenation states.
5. Identify appropriate nursing interventions for a patient admitted with pneumonia and emphysema.
6. Identify appropriate discharge teaching needs for a patient with altered oxygenation.

In this lesson you will learn the essentials of caring for a patient diagnosed with pneumonia and emphysema. You will explore the patient's history, evaluate presenting symptoms and treatment on admission, and assess the patient's progress throughout the hospital stay. Patricia Newman is a 61-year-old female admitted with pneumonia and a history of emphysema. Begin this lesson by reviewing the general concepts of emphysema and pneumonia as presented in your textbook.

Exercise 1

✎ **Clinical Preparation: Writing Activity**

🕐 20 minutes

1. What category of lung diseases does emphysema belong to?

• Click on **Go to Nurses' Station**.
- Click on **Chart** and then on **406**.
- Click on **History and Physical**.

3. What risk factors for community-acquired pneumonia does Patricia Newman have?

 • Click on **Return to Nurses' Station**.
- Click on **406** to enter Patricia Newman's room.
- Read the **Initial Observations**.

4. What would be your priority nursing assessment/intervention(s) based on your initial observations of this patient?

 • Click on **Patient Care**. Perform a focused assessment based on her admitting diagnosis.

5. Record your findings below. How has Patricia Newman's condition changed since report?

Focused Assessment Area	Assessment Findings	Change in Assessment
Respiratory		
Cardiovascular		
Mental Status		

• Click on **Nurse-Client Interactions**.
   • Select and view the video titiled **0730: Prioritizing Interventions**. (*Note:* If this video title is not available, check the virtual clock to see whether enough time has elapsed. The video cannot be viewed before its specified time.)

   6. Evaluate the nurse's actions based on the patient's current status. How does this nurse's action differ from your plan of care as answered in question 4?

 7. What nursing interventions would be appropriate to improve Patricia Newman's airway clearance and gas exchange? (*Hint:* See page 627 in your textbook.)

   • Click on **Chart** and then on **406**.
   • Click on **Laboratory Reports**.

   8. Identify any abnormal lab results and describe how they correlate with Patricia Newman's diagnosis of pneumonia.

→ • Click on **Return to Room 406**.
  • Click on **MAR** and then on tab **406**.

9. What is the desired therapeutic effect of ipratropium bromide? How could the nurse assess whether the desired effect was achieved?

10. What is the desired therapeutic effect of cefotetan? How could the nurse assess whether the desired effect was achieved?

11. What is the rationale for administration of IV fluids related to pneumonia?

→ • Click on **Medication Room**.
  • Click on **MAR** to determine medications that Patricia Newman is ordered to receive at 0800 and any appropriate prn medications you may want to administer. (*Note:* You may click on **Review MAR** at any time to verify correct medication order. Remember to look at the patient name on the MAR to make sure you have the correct patient's record—you must click on the correct room number within the MAR. Click on **Return to Medication Room** after reviewing the correct MAR.)
  • Click on **Unit Dosage**. When the close-up view appears, click on drawer **406**.
  • Select the medication(s) you plan to administer. After each medication you select, click **Put Medication on Tray**. When you are finished, click on **Close Drawer**.
  • Click **View Medication Room**.
  • Click on **IV Storage**. From the close-up view, click on the drawer labeled **Large Volume**.
  • Select the medication(s) you plan to administer, put medication(s) on tray, and close bin.
  • Click **View Medication Room**.
  • Click on **Preparation**. Select the correct medication to administer; click **Prepare** and **Next**.
  • Choose the correct patient to administer this medication to and click **Finish**.
  • Repeat the above two steps until all medications that you want to administer are prepared.
  • You can click **Review Your Medications** and then **Return to Medication Room** when ready. From the Medication Room, you may go directly to Patricia Newman's room by clicking on **406** at bottom of screen.

- Administer the medication, utilizing the five rights of medication administration. After you have collected the appropriate assessment data and are ready for administration, click **Patient Care** and then **Medication Administration**. Verify that the correct patient and medication(s) appear in the left-hand window. Then click the down arrow next to Select. From the drop-down menu, select **Administer** and complete the Administration Wizard by providing any information requested. When the Wizard stops asking for information, click **Administer to Patient**. Specify **Yes** when asked whether this administration should be recorded in the MAR. Finally, click **Finish**.

Now let's see how you did!

→ • Click on **Leave the Floor** at the bottom of your screen. From the Floor Menu, select **Look at Your Preceptor's Evaluation**. Then click on **Medication Scorecard**.

12. Note below whether or not you correctly administered the appropriate medications. If not, why do you think you were incorrect? According to Table C in this scorecard, what are the appropriate resources that should be used and important assessments that should be completed before administering these medications? Did you use these resources and perform these assessments correctly?

Exercise 3

CD-ROM Activity

40 minutes

- Sign in to work at Pacific View Regional Hospital for Period of Care 2. (*Note:* If you are already in the virtual hospital from a previous exercise, click on **Leave the Floor** and then **Restart the Program** to get to the sign-in window.)
- From the Patient List, select Patricia Newman (Room 406).
- Click on **Go to Nurses' Station**.
- Click on **Chart** and then on **406**.
- Click on **History and Physical**.

1. How long has Patricia Newman been diagnosed with emphysema?

11. What do you think her special dietary needs are? Give a rationale for your answer.

12. What is educational goal 6 for Patricia Newman?

 13. Explain the rationale for using this technique. How would you teach this patient to cough effectively? (*Hint:* See page 627 in your textbook.)

 14. Since Patricia Newman's emphysema puts her at high risk for pulmonary infections, what would you teach her to do to help prevent further episodes of pneumonia? (*Hint:* See page 628 in your textbook.)

→ • Click on **Return to Nurses' Station**.
  • Click on **406** to go to Patricia Newman's room.
  • Click on **Patient Care**.
  • Click on **Nurse-Client Interactions**.
  • Select and view the video titled **1100: Care Coordination**.

15. What disciplines are involved in planning and providing care for Patricia Newman? List these in the left column below. In the right column, explain the role of each person in helping meet the patient's health care needs.

Involved Disciplines   **Role in Patricia Newman's Health Care**

Asthma

Reading Assignment: Lower Airway Problems (Chapter 26)

Patient: Jacquline Catanazaro, Room 402

Goal: Utilize the nursing process to competently care for patients with asthma.

Objectives:

1. Identify clinical manifestations of an acute asthmatic exacerbation.
2. Evaluate diagnostic tests as they relate to a patient's oxygenation status.
3. Describe medications used to treat asthma, including mechanism of action and therapeutic effects.
4. Prioritize nursing care for a patient with an acute exacerbation of asthma.
5. Formulate an appropriate patient education plan regarding home asthma management for a patient with identified barriers to learning.

In this lesson you will learn the essentials of caring for a patient diagnosed with asthma. You will explore the patient's history, evaluate presenting symptoms and treatment on admission, and follow the patient's progress throughout the hospital stay. Jacquline Catanazaro is a 45-year-old female admitted with increasing respiratory distress. Begin this lesson by reviewing the general concepts of asthma as presented in your textbook.

Exercise 1

Clinical Preparation: Writing Activity

30 minutes

1. What is another name for asthma?

2. What pathologic triggers can lead to an exacerbation of asthma?

3. Does Jacquline Catanazaro's history identify any of these triggers?

4. What other factor(s) might be contributing to her asthma exacerbations?

5. Based on her history and home medication regimen, what step of asthma management do you think she is normally at (excluding this admission for an exacerbation)? Explain.

⟶ • Click on **Emergency Department**.

6. What were Jacquline Catanazaro's presenting symptoms?

7. What diagnostic testing was ordered? Document and interpret the abnormal results below. (*Hint:* Review the Laboratory Reports and Diagnostic Reports sections of the chart to obtain these results.)

8. Read the ED physician's progress notes for 1400. What are the results of the patient's PEFR? How would you interpret these in light of her present condition?

 • Click on **Physician's Orders**.

9. What medical treatment is ordered in the ED? (*Hint:* See orders for Monday at 1005.)

10. How would you evaluate the patient's response to medical treatment?

11. What medications were ordered on Monday at 1600? What is the mechanism of action for each of these drugs? (*Hint:* Click on **Return to Nurses' Station**; then click on the **Drug** icon in the lower left corner of your screen.)

12. In what order would the nurse administer these medications? Explain.

13. What new medications are ordered on Tuesday at 0800? Provide a rationale for these orders. Why is the prednisone ordered to be decreased by 5 mg every day?

Exercise 3

 CD-ROM Activity

30 minutes

- Sign in to work at Pacific View Regional Hospital for Period of Care 1. (*Note:* If you are already in the virtual hospital from a previous exercise, click on **Leave the Floor** and then **Restart the Program** to get to the sign-in window.)
- From the Patient List, select Jacquline Catanazaro (Room 402).
- Click on **Go to Nurses' Station**.
- Click on **402**.
- Click on **Initial Observations**.

1. Describe your initial observations when you enter Jacquline Catanazaro's room.

→ • Click on **Take Vital Signs**.

2. Record Jacquline Catanazaro's vital signs below.

3. Are there any clinical alerts for Jacquline Catanazaro? If so, describe below.

4. How would you prioritize your care for her at this point?

→ • Click on **Patient Care**.

5. Perform and document a focused assessment on three priority areas, based on Jacquline Catanazaro's present status.

Focused Areas of Assessment	Jacquline Catanazaro's Assessment Findings

 • Click on **Chart** and then on **402**.
   • Click on **Physician's Orders**.

6. What new orders did the physician write on Monday at 0730?

 • Click on **Return to Room 402**.
   • Click on **Nurse-Client Interactions**.
   • Select and view the video titled **0730: Intervention—Anxiety**. (*Note:* If this video title is not available, check the virtual clock to see whether enough time has elapsed. The video cannot be viewed before its specified time.)

7. How does this nurse prioritize her actions? Give a rationale for these actions?

 • Click on **Clinical Alerts**.

8. Look at the 0800 clinical alert. Interpret this alert below.

 • Click on **Chart** and then on **402**.
   • Click on **Physician's Notes**.

9. Read the notes for Wednesday at 0800. How does the physician evaluate the patient's condition at this point?

 • Click on **Physician's Orders**. Find the orders for 0800 on Wednesday.

10. Record the orders for 0800 on Wednesday below. Provide a rationale or expected therapeutic response for each.

New Orders   **Rationale/Expected Therapeutic Response**

Exercise 4

 CD-ROM Activity

 45 minutes

- Sign in to work at Pacific View Regional Hospital for Period of Care 2. (*Note:* If you are already in the virtual hospital from a previous exercise, click on **Leave the Floor** and then **Restart the Program** to get to the sign-in window.)
- From the Patient List, select Jacquline Catanazaro (Room 402).
- Click on **Get Report**.

1. Briefly summarize the activity for Jacquline Catanazaro over the last 4 hours.

- Click on **Go to Nurses' Station**.
- Click on **402** to go to the patient's room.

2. What is your initial observation of Jacquline Catanazaro for this time period?

3. Are there any clinical alerts?

- Click on **Take Vital Signs**.

4. Record Jacquline Catanazaro's current vital signs below. How do these results compare with those you obtained during Period of Care 1? (*Hint:* See Exercise 3, question 2 of this lesson.)

• Click on **Patient Care**.

5. Perform a focused assessment on Jacquline Catanazaro. Record your findings in the middle column below. In the last column, compare these findings with those you obtained during Period of Care 1. Interpret your results. (*Hint:* See Exercise 3, question 5.)

Focused Areas of Assessment	Current Findings	Comparison with 0800 Findings—Interpretation of Results

 • Click on **Nurse-Client Interactions**.
   • Select and view the video titled **1115: Assessment—Readiness to Learn**. (*Note:* If this video title is not available, check the virtual clock to see whether enough time has elapsed. The video cannot be viewed before its specified time.)

6. Describe the nurse's actions. Are they appropriate? Explain.

7. What barriers to learning might be present for Jacquline Catanazaro?

→ • Click on **Leave the Floor**.
   • Click on **Restart the Program**.
   • Sign in to work at Pacific View Regional Hospital for Period of Care 3.
   • From the Patient List, select Jacquline Catanazaro (Room 402).
   • Click on **Go to Nurses' Station**.
   • Click on **402**.
   • Click on **Patient Care**.
   • Click on **Nurse-Client Interactions**.
   • Select and view the video titled **1500: Intervention—Patient Teaching**. (*Note:* If this video title is not available, check the virtual clock to see whether enough time has elapsed. The video cannot be viewed before its specified time.)

8. In the video, what equipment is the nurse teaching the patient about?

9. What should Jacquline Catanazaro be taught regarding the results of her peak flow measurements?

10. Document directions you would give Jacquline Catanazaro for properly using a metered dose inhaler (MDI).

11. What other asthma management needs would you teach this patient?

→ • Click on **Chart** and then on **402** for Jacquline Catanazaro's record.
  • Click on **Patient Education**.

12. What are the educational goals for Jacquline Catanazaro?

13. Describe the differences in outcomes met for Jacquline Catanazaro and her sister.

14. The patient is scheduled for discharge tomorrow. Do you have any concerns? What would be your most appropriate action?

LESSON **12** _____

Atrial Fibrillation

/OO **Reading Assignment:** Assessment of the Cardiovascular System (Chapter 28)
Coronary Artery Disease and Dysrhythmias (Chapter 29)

Patients: Piya Jordan, Room 403

Goal: Utilize the nursing process to competently care for patients with dysrhythmias.

Objectives:

1. Describe telemetry rhythm strip characteristics of atrial fibrillation.
2. Identify potential etiologic causes of atrial fibrillation for an assigned patient.
3. Assess a patient for clinical manifestations of atrial fibrillation.
4. Develop a plan of care to monitor a patient for potential complications of atrial fibrillation.
5. Perform appropriate assessments prior to administering pharmacologic therapy for atrial fibrillation.
6. Accurately administer IV digoxin.
7. Discuss the use of anticoagulation therapy for a patient with atrial fibrillation.
8. Develop appropriate educational outcomes for a patient with a history of atrial fibrillation.

In this lesson you will learn the essentials of caring for a patient with a cardiac dysrhythmia. You will explore the patient's history, evaluate presenting symptoms and treatment, provide appropriate nursing interventions, and plan an appropriate patient educational outcome related to the dysrhythmia. Piya Jordan is a 68-year-old female admitted with nausea, vomiting, and abdominal pain.

Exercise 1

 Clinical Preparation: Writing Activity

20 minutes

1. Briefly describe the three pathophysiologic mechanisms that can cause dysrhythmias.

2. Descibe the concept of *atrial kick*. Why is this important? (*Hint:* See page 714 in your text-book.)

3. Identify the cardiac event represented by each of the following waves and measured intervals.

   a. P wave

   b. QRS wave

   c. T wave

   d. PR interval

e. ST segment

f. QT interval

g. U wave

4. Describe the seven steps of ECG analysis.

a.

b.

c.

d.

e.

f.

g.

10. Did Piya Jordan have a 12-lead ECG done? If yes, what was the rhythm? If not, do you think it should have been done? Why or why not?

11. For what potential complications should you monitor Piya Jordan?

Exercise 3

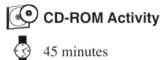 **CD-ROM Activity**

45 minutes

- Sign in to work at Pacific View Regional Hospital for Period of Care 1. (*Note:* If you are already in the virtual hospital from a previous exercise, click on **Leave the Floor** and then **Restart the Program** to get to the sign-in window.)
- From the Patient List, select Piya Jordan (Room 403).
- Click on **Go to Nurses' Station**.
- Click on **MAR** and then select tab **403**.

1. What medication is prescribed to treat Piya Jordan's atrial fibrillation? Describe the pharmacodynamics of this medication as related to atrial fibrillation. (*Hint:* You may need to consult the Drug Guide.)

2. Why did the physician order a digoxin level when the patient first presented to the ED? (*Hint:* Review her presenting symptoms, as well as the Drug Guide.)

• Click on **Return to Nurses' Station**.
   • Click on **Chart** and then on **403**.
   • Click on **Laboratory Reports**.

   3. What was the digoxin level? Is this therapeutic or toxic?

   4. For what other symptoms would you monitor Piya Jordan in relation to digoxin toxicity?

 • Click on **History and Physical**.

   5. What other medication was prescribed for Piya Jordan related to atrial fibrillation prior to this admission? Explain the rationale for this medication. (*Hint:* Think of potential serious complications of atrial fibrillation.)

 • Click on **Physician's Orders**.

   6. What two items did the physician prescribe preoperatively to reverse Piya Jordan's anti-coagulation? How would you know whether this was effective? Please explain.

7. What was ordered postoperatively to prevent clot formation?

 • Click on **Nursing Admission**.

8. What knowledge (or lack of knowledge) does Piya Jordan verbalize regarding her history of atrial fibrillation? (*Hint:* Check the Health Promotion section.)

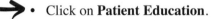 • Click on **Patient Education**.

9. What might you add to these outcomes based on your answer to question 8?

10. What other treatment options are available to treat Piya Jordan's atrial fibrillation?

11. What interventional therapy may be used for patients with recurrent or sustained atrial fibrillation?

→ • Click on **Return to Nurses' Station**.

• Click on **Medication Room**.

• Click on **MAR** to determine medications that Piya Jordan is ordered to receive at 0800. (*Note:* You may click on **Review MAR** at any time to verify correct medication order. Remember to look at the patient name on the MAR to make sure you have the correct patient's record—you must click on the correct room number within the MAR. Click on **Return to Medication Room** after reviewing the correct MAR.)

• Based on your care for Piya Jordan, access the various storage areas of the Medication Room to obtain the necessary medications you need to administer.

• For each area you access, first select the medication you plan to administer, then click **Put Medication on Tray**. When finished with a storage area, click on **Close Drawer**.

• Click **View Medication Room**.

• Click on **Preparation** and choose the correct medication to administer. Click **Prepare**.

• Click **Next** and choose the correct patient to administer this medication to. Click **Finish**.

• Repeat the above two steps until all medications that you want to administer are prepared.

• You can click **Review Your Medications** and then **Return to Medication Room** when you are ready. Once you are back in the Medication Room, you may go directly to Piya Jordan's room by clicking on **403** at the bottom of the screen.

• Administer the medication, utilizing the five rights of medication administration. After you have collected the appropriate assessment data and are ready for administration, click **Patient Care** and then **Medication Administration**. Verify that the correct patient and medication(s) appear in the left-hand window. Then click the down arrow next to Select. From the drop-down menu, select **Administer** and complete the Administration Wizard by providing any information requested. When the Wizard stops asking for information, click **Administer to Patient**. Specify **Yes** when asked whether this administration should be recorded in the MAR. Finally, click **Finish**.

12. Over how many minutes would you administer the IV digoxin?

13. What should you have assessed before administering digoxin to Piya Jordan today?

Exercise 1

Clinical Preparation: Writing Activity

20 minutes

1. Identify and describe the classifications of blood pressure as presented in your textbook. (*Hint:* See pages 859-861 in your textbook.)

2. Identify and describe four physiologic controls of blood pressure.

   a.

   b.

c.

d.

3. Define the following terms.

   a. Primary (essential) hypertension

   b. Secondary hypertension

4. List the risk factors for primary (essential) hypertension. (*Hint:* See page 859 in your text-book.)

   a.

   b.

   c.

   d.

   e.

   f.

   g.

   h.

Exercise 2

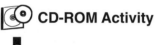 **CD-ROM Activity**

 45 minutes

- Sign in to work at Pacific View Regional Hospital for Period of Care 1. (*Note:* If you are already in the virtual hospital from a previous exercise, click on **Leave the Floor** and then **Restart the Program** to get to the sign-in window.)
- From the Patient List, select Patricia Newman (Room 406).
- Click on **Go to Nurses' Station**.
- Click on **Chart** and then on **406**.
- Click on **History and Physical**.

   1. How long has Patricia Newman been diagnosed with hypertension?

→ • Click on **Nursing Admission**.

   2. What risk factors for hypertension does she have?

→ • Click on **Physician's Orders**.

3. In the left column below, list all medications ordered to treat Patricia Newman's hypertension. For each medication, identify the drug classification and mechanism of action. (*Note:* You will complete the table in questions 4 and 5.)

Medication	Drug Classification	Mechanism of Action	Nursing Assessments	Side Effects

• Click on **Nursing Admission**.

13. Was Patricia Newman following any of the interventions you identified in question 12 to reduce her blood pressure at home? Explain.

 • Click on **Physician's Orders**.

14. Identify any of the interventions addressed in question 12 that were ordered for this patient during this hospital stay.

15. As the nurse caring for Patricia Newman, what do you think would be your professional responsibility related to your findings for questions 13 and 14?

Exercise 3

 CD-ROM Activity

40 minutes

- Sign in to work at Pacific View Regional Hospital for Period of Care 1. (*Note:* If you are already in the virtual hospital from a previous exercise, click on **Leave the Floor** and then **Restart the Program** to get to the sign-in window.)
- From the Patient List, select Harry George (Room 401).
- Click on **Go to Nurses' Station**.
- Click on **EPR** and then on **Login**.
- Select **401** for the patient's room and **Vital Signs** as the category.

1. Document Harry George's blood pressure results below.

	Tues 0305	Tues 0705	Tues 1105	Tues 1505	Tues 1905	Tues 2305	Wed 0305	Wed 0705
Blood pressure								

 • Click on **Exit EPR**.
- Click on **Chart** and then on **401**.
- Click on **History and Physical**.

2. Does Harry George have a history of hypertension?

3. Does he have any risk factors for hypertension? If yes, please identify.

4. Based on the blood pressure recordings in question 1, in what classification would you put Harry George's blood pressure?

5. For what potential complications should you assess Harry George related to untreated hypertension?

 • Click on **Physician's Orders**.

6. Several diagnostic tests were ordered by the physician. Although these tests may have been ordered for various purposes, they may specifically help to identify target organ disease. In the middle column below, indicate how each test might be helpful. (*Hint:* You may refer to a laboratory/diagnostic reference manual for help. You will complete this table in questions 7 and 8.)

Diagnostic Test	How Test Might Help Identify Target Organ Disease	Results
Chest x-ray		
BUN		
Creatinine		
Urinalysis		

 • Click on **Diagnostic Reports**.

7. Record the result of the chest x-ray in the third column of the table above and indicate whether the results suggest the presence of target organ disease.

 • Click on **Laboratory Reports**.

8. Find and record the lab results for BUN, creatinine, and urinalysis in the table above. Indicate what these results mean related to target organ disease.

9. In the table below, identify the various classifications of hypertensive medication that might be used to treat Harry George's elevated blood pressure. For each classification, briefly describe the mechanism of action.

Drug Classification	Mechanism of Action
a.	
b.	
c.	
d.	
e.	
f.	
g.	
h.	
i.	
j.	
k.	
l.	

10. What symptoms might Harry George display if his diastolic blood pressure dramatically increased above 130 mm Hg?

11. What specific measurement is used to assess the seriousness of the patient's condition in hypertensive crisis?

12. Describe the collaborative management of a patient with a hypertensive emergency.

DVT and Pulmonary Embolism

⌇✍ **Reading Assignment:**   Lower Airway Problems (Chapter 26)
Vascular Problems (Chapter 31)

Patient: Clarence Hughes, Room 404

Goal: Utilize the nursing process to competently care for patients with a critically altered oxygenation state.

Objectives:

1. Identify clinical manifestations of pulmonary embolism.
2. Prioritize nursing care for a patient with acute onset of respiratory distress and chest pain.
3. Describe diagnostic testing relative to the diagnosis of pulmonary embolism.
4. Describe pharmacologic therapy for a patient with a pulmonary embolism.
5. Accurately calculate correct dosage of heparin for a patient using a sliding scale.
6. Identify disease management issues regarding the care of a patient with a pulmonary embolism.

In this lesson you will learn the essentials of caring for a patient diagnosed with an acute pulmonary embolism as a sequalae of deep vein thrombosis. You will explore the patient's history, evaluate presenting symptoms and treatment, provide appropriate nursing interventions, and assess the patient's progress throughout the clinical day. Clarence Hughes is a 73-year-old male admitted for an elective left knee arthroplasty.

Exercise 1

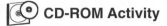 **CD-ROM Activity**

30 minutes

- Sign in to work at Pacific View Regional Hospital for Period of Care 2. (*Note:* If you are already in the virtual hospital from a previous exercise, click on **Leave the Floor** and then **Restart the Program** to get to the sign-in window.)
- From the Patient List, select Clarence Hughes (Room 404).
- Click on **Get Report**.

1. Before entering Clarence Hughes' room, summarize what you would expect to find based on the report you just received.

- Click on **Go to Nurses' Station**.
- Click on **404** to go to the patient's room

2. What is your initial observation as you enter the patient's room?

3. What should your priority actions be at this point?

- Click on **Patient Care**.
- Click on **Nurse-Client Interactions**.
- Select and view the video titled **1115: Interventions—Airway**. (*Note:* If this video title is not available, check the virtual clock to see whether enough time has elapsed. The video cannot be viewed before its specified time.)

4. Describe the nurse's actions in this video. Should the nurse have left the patient to go get oxygen? Explain your answer. If not, what else could she have done?

5. What signs of pulmonary embolism is Clarence Hughes displaying?

6. Suspecting a pulmonary embolism, for what other clinical manifestations would you assess Clarence Hughes?

 • Click on **Chart** and then on **404**.
   • Click on **History and Physical**.

7. Based on the patient's history and current reason for hospitalization, what risk factors for DVT and resultant pulmonary embolism does Clarence Hughes have?

• Click on **Physician's Orders**.

8. Look at the orders for Wednesday at 1120. Document these orders below and provide a rationale for each.

Physician's Order	Rationale

➡ • Click on **Return to Room 404**.
   • Click on **Patient Care** and then on **Nurse-Client Interactions**.
   • Select and view the video titled **1135: Change in Patient Condition**. (*Note:* If this video title is not available, check the virtual clock to see whether enough time has elapsed. The video cannot be viewed before its specified time.)

9. As the nurse is explaining care to the family, she states that a transporter will be coming to take the Clarence Hughes for a ventilation-perfusion scan. Would you send this patient down to radiology with just the transporter? Why or why not?

Exercise 2

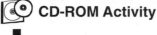 **CD-ROM Activity**

30 minutes

- Sign in to work at Pacific View Regional Hospital for Period of Care 3. (*Note:* If you are already in the virtual hospital from a previous exercise, click on **Leave the Floor** and then **Restart the Program** to get to the sign-in window.)
- From the Patient List, select Clarence Hughes (Room 404).
- Click on **Go to Nurses' Station**.
- Click on **Chart** and then on **404**.
- Select and review the **Laboratory Reports** and **Diagnostic Reports** sections of the chart.

1. Document the results of the diagnostic testing ordered for Clarence Hughes.

Diagnostic Test	Result

- Click on **Physician's Orders**.

2. What orders were written to treat Clarence Hughes' pulmonary embolism?

3. What lab test will be used to titrate the heparin infusion? What are the normal values for this test?

4. What is the desired therapeutic level for this test? (*Hint:* You may consult the Drug Guide in the Nurses' Station.)

 • Click on **Return to Nurses' Station**.
   • Click on **MAR** and then on **404** for Clarence Hughes' record.

5. How many mL of heparin would you administer for the bolus dose?

6. If you were the nurse starting the heparin infusion, at what rate would you set the IV pump to infuse this medication?

 • Click on **Return to Nurses' Station**.
   • Click on **Chart** and then on **404**.
   • Click on **Laboratory Reports**.

7. What were the results of the aPTT and INR at 1300 today? Why were these tests ordered prior to starting the heparin?

 • Click on **Return to Nurses' Station**.
   • Click on **404** to enter Clarence Hughes' room.
   • Click on **Patient Care** and then on **Patient-Client Interactions**.
   • Select and view the video titled **1510: Disease Management**. (*Note:* If this video title is not available, check the virtual clock to see whether enough time has elapsed. The video cannot be viewed before its specified time.)

8. When the son asks the nurse whether the pulmonary embolism would delay his father's discharge, the nurse states that the heparin takes two days to stabilize. Does this mean that the patient will be discharged on heparin? If not, what medication will be used to minimize clot formation? Explain why the patient is not started on this medication rather than heparin.

9. What lab test(s) will be used to monitor the therapeutic effect of coumadin? What is the therapeutic range for these tests?

10. For what possible complications would you monitor Clarence Hughes related to the pulmonary embolism? (*Hint:* See pages 662-665 in your textbook.)

Exercise 3

CD-ROM Activity

30 minutes

- Sign in to work at Pacific View Regional Hospital for Period of Care 4. (*Note:* If you are already in the virtual hospital from a previous exercise, click on **Leave the Floor** and then **Restart the Program** to get to the sign-in window.)
- From the Patient List, select Clarence Hughes (Room 404).
- Click on **Go to Nurses' Station**.
- Click on **Chart** and then on **404**.
- Click on **Laboratory Report**.

1. What is the aPTT result for 1900?

- Click on **Return to Nurses' Station**.
- Click on **MAR** and then on tab **404**.

2. What would you do now with the heparin infusion? Calculate the correct infusion rate and document below. (*Hint:* Refer to your answer for question 6 in Exercise 2.)

➡ • Click on **Return to Nurses' Station**.
  • Click on **Kardex** and choose tab **404**. Review the stated outcomes for Clarence Hughes.

3. Are there any additional outcomes that should be added based on his current setback? Explain.

4. If the heparin is not effective in treating Clarence Hughes and/or his condition worsens, what other pharmacologic treatment might be helpful? Explain.

5. Describe bleeding precautions that must be followed while Clarence Hughes is receiving heparin therapy. Explain.

6. If Clarence Hughes' condition deteriorates, what surgical treatment would be needed? Explain.

 7. If Clarence Hughes develops another pulmonary embolism while being treated with anticoagulation therapy, what further treatment might the physician consider to prevent the recurrence of PEs? Explain. (*Hint:* See pages 888-889 in your textbook.)

➤ • Click on **Return to Nurses' Station**.
  • Click on **403** to enter Piya Jordan's room.
  • Click on **Patient Care**.
  • Click on **Nurse-Client Interaction**.
  • Select and view the video titled **0735: Pain—Adverse Drug Event**. (*Note:* If this video title is not available, check the virtual clock to see whether enough time has elapsed. The video cannot be viewed before its specified time.)

4. What does the nurse state she will do to prepare the patient for a blood transfusion?

5. What gauge IV would you insert for the blood transfusion?

6. What other pretransfusion responsibilities would you complete? Have these been completed? (*Hint:* Check the patient's chart.)

➤ • Click on **Chart** and then on **403**.
  • Click on **Laboratory Reports**.

7. What day and time was the cross-match completed? Is this lab result acceptable for blood being transfused today?

8. Explain how you would prepare the blood set-up prior to administration.

LESSON 15

Blood Component Therapy

✎ **Reading Assignment:** Assessment of the Hematologic System (Chapter 32)
Hematologic Problems (Chapter 33)

Patient: Piya Jordan, Room 403

Goal: Utilize the nursing process to competently care for patients receiving various blood products.

Objectives:

1. Describe the ABO and Rh antigen systems.
2. Identify the correct blood type to administer to a specific patient.
3. Describe appropriate nursing responsibilities related to blood product administration.
4. Evaluate vital sign assessments related to potential blood transfusion reactions.
5. Describe appropriate assessment parameters when monitoring for various types of transfusion reactions.

In this lesson you will learn the essentials of caring for a patient receiving blood and blood product transfusions. You will describe pretransfusion responsibilities, identify administration specifics, and evaluate the patient during and after each transfusion. Piya Jordan is a 68-year-old female admitted with nausea, vomiting, and abdominal pain.

Exercise 1

Clinical Preparation: Writing Activity

10 minutes

1. Describe the ABO antigen system.

2. Describe the Rh antigen system.

3. Complete the table below to identify which types of blood are compatible with each other.

Patient's Blood Type	Blood Types That This Patient Can Receive
A+	
A–	
B+	
B–	
O+	
O–	
AB+	
AB–	

Exercise 2

CD-ROM Activity

30 minutes

- Sign in to work at Pacific View Regional Hospital for Period of Care 1. (*Note:* If you are already in the virtual hospital from a previous exercise, click on **Leave the Floor** and then **Restart the Program** to get to the sign-in window.)
- From the Patient List, select Piya Jordan (Room 403).
- Click on **Go to Nurses' Station**.
- Click on **Chart** and then on **403**.
- Click on **Laboratory Reports**.

1. Document the results of Piya Jordan's hematology results below.

	Monday 2200	Tuesday 0630	Wednesday 063
Hemoglobin			
Hematocrit			

2. Why do you think her H&H is lower on Wednesday? (*Hint:* Check the Physican's Notes in the chart.)

- Click on **Physician's Orders**.

3. What was ordered to correct this? Is this appropriate related to Piya Jordan's level of hemoglobin? Explain why or why not.

LESSON 15 ——————————————————————

Blood Component Therapy

———————————————————————————

Reading Assignment: Assessment of the Hematologic System (Chapter 32)
Hematologic Problems (Chapter 33)

Patient: Piya Jordan, Room 403

Goal: Utilize the nursing process to competently care for patients receiving various blood products.

Objectives:

1. Describe the ABO and Rh antigen systems.
2. Identify the correct blood type to administer to a specific patient.
3. Describe appropriate nursing responsibilities related to blood product administration.
4. Evaluate vital sign assessments related to potential blood transfusion reactions.
5. Describe appropriate assessment parameters when monitoring for various types of transfusion reactions.

In this lesson you will learn the essentials of caring for a patient receiving blood and blood product transfusions. You will describe pretransfusion responsibilities, identify administration specifics, and evaluate the patient during and after each transfusion. Piya Jordan is a 68-year-old female admitted with nausea, vomiting, and abdominal pain.

Exercise 1

 Clinical Preparation: Writing Activity

10 minutes

1. Describe the ABO antigen system.

2. Describe the Rh antigen system.

3. Complete the table below to identify which types of blood are compatible with each other.

Patient's Blood Type	Blood Types That This Patient Can Receive
A+	
A–	
B+	
B–	
O+	
O–	
AB+	
AB–	

Exercise 2

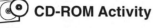 **CD-ROM Activity**

30 minutes

- Sign in to work at Pacific View Regional Hospital for Period of Care 1. (*Note:* If you are already in the virtual hospital from a previous exercise, click on **Leave the Floor** and then **Restart the Program** to get to the sign-in window.)
- From the Patient List, select Piya Jordan (Room 403).
- Click on **Go to Nurses' Station**.
- Click on **Chart** and then on **403**.
- Click on **Laboratory Reports**.

1. Document the results of Piya Jordan's hematology results below.

	Monday 2200	Tuesday 0630	Wednesday 0630
Hemoglobin			
Hematocrit			

2. Why do you think her H&H is lower on Wednesday? (*Hint:* Check the Physician's Notes in the chart.)

 • Click on **Physician's Orders**.

3. What was ordered to correct this? Is this appropriate related to Piya Jordan's level of hemoglobin? Explain why or why not.

→ • Click on **Return to Nurses' Station**.
- Click on **403** to enter Piya Jordan's room.
- Click on **Patient Care**.
- Click on **Nurse-Client Interaction**.
- Select and view the video titled **0735: Pain—Adverse Drug Event**. (*Note:* If this video title is not available, check the virtual clock to see whether enough time has elapsed. The video cannot be viewed before its specified time.)

4. What does the nurse state she will do to prepare the patient for a blood transfusion?

5. What gauge IV would you insert for the blood transfusion?

6. What other pretransfusion responsibilities would you complete? Have these been completed? (*Hint:* Check the patient's chart.)

→ • Click on **Chart** and then on **403**.
- Click on **Laboratory Reports**.

7. What day and time was the cross-match completed? Is this lab result acceptable for blood being transfused today?

8. Explain how you would prepare the blood set-up prior to administration.

Exercise 3

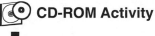 **CD-ROM Activity**

30 minutes

- Sign in to work at Pacific View Regional Hospital for Period of Care 2. (*Note:* If you are already in the virtual hospital from a previous exercise, click on **Leave the Floor** and then **Restart the Program** to get to the sign-in window.)
- From the Patient List, select Piya Jordan (Room 403).
- Click on **Go to Nurses' Station** and then on **403** to enter Piya Jordan's room.
- First, select **Patient Care**; then click on **Nurse-Client Interactions**.
- Select and view the video titled **1115: Interventions—Nausea and Blood**. (*Note:* If this video title is not available, check the virtual clock to see whether enough time has elapsed. The video cannot be viewed before its specified time.)

1. Piya Jordan's daughter verbalizes concern regarding the safety of blood transfusion. How did the nurse respond to this?

2. Describe how you would explain the safety of blood transfusions.

3. During the video, the nurse states that the blood has just arrived. How soon should the nurse begin the transfusion?

→ - Click on **Chart** and then on **403**.
- Click on **Laboratory Reports**.

4. What is Piya Jordan's blood type?

5. What type of blood may she receive safely?

6. Describe the nurse's responsibilities during the initiation of this transfusion.

7. How fast would you transfuse this unit of blood? Give your rationale.

8. What assessments should be completed on Piya Jordan during the transfusion?

9. What would you document regarding this blood transfusion?

Exercise 4

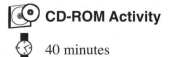 **CD-ROM Activity**

40 minutes

- Sign in to work at Pacific View Regional Hospital for Period of Care 4. (*Note:* If you are already in the virtual hospital from a previous exercise, click on **Leave the Floor** and then **Restart the Program** to get to the sign-in window.)
- From the Patient List, select Piya Jordan (Room 403).
- Click on **Go to Nurses' Station**; then click on **EPR** and **Login**.
- Choose **403** from the Patient drop-down menu; select **Vital Signs** as the category.

1. Below, document Piya Jordan's vital signs as recorded in the EPR after each of the two units of blood.

	1130	1145	1200	1215	1315	1400
Temp						
Pulse						
BP						
Resp						

	1415	1430	1445	1500	1515	1530
Temp						
Pulse						
BP						
Resp						

2. According to the vital signs you recorded in question 1, did Piya Jordan have any adverse reactions to the blood transfusions? Explain.

3. What type of symptoms would you expect to see if she had a hemolytic transfusion reaction?

LESSON 16

Diabetes Mellitus, Part 1

∽ **Reading Assignment:** Diabetes Mellitus and Hypoglycemia (Chapter 39)

Patients: Harry George, Room 401

Goal: Utilize the nursing process to competently care for patients with diabetes mellitus.

Objectives:

1. Describe the etiology of type 1 and type 2 diabetes mellitus.
2. Compare and contrast the characteristics of type 1 and type 2 diabetes.
3. Identify the relationship between diabetes and other disease processes.
4. Evaluate a patient's risk factors for diabetes.
5. Assess a patient for short- and long-term complications of diabetes.
6. Develop an appropriate plan of care for a patient with type 2 diabetes.

In this lesson you will learn the essentials of caring for a patient admitted with complications related to diabetes mellitus. You will explore the patient's history, evaluate presenting symptoms and treatment, plan appropriate nursing interventions, and develop an individualized teaching plan. Harry George is a 54-year-old male with a 4-year history of type 2 diabetes, admitted with infection and swelling of his left foot.

Exercise 1

Clinical Preparation: Writing Activity

20 minutes

1. Briefly define and summarize the etiologic differences between type 1 and type 2 diabetes mellitus.

Type 1 diabetes mellitus

Type 2 diabetes mellitus

2. Compare and contrast the distinquishing characteristics of type 1 and type 2 diabetes mellitus (DM) by completing the table below.

Features	Type 1 DM	Type 2 DM
Age at onset		
Type of onset		
Clinical presentation/ symptoms		
Endogenous insulin		
Prevalance		
Islet cell antibodies		
Environmental factors		
Medications		
Nutritional status		
Vascular and neurolgic complications		

1. What test is ordered that can be used to determine Harry George's control of diabetes mellitus? Describe the purpose of this test.

2. What was the result of this test for Harry George? Evaluate and explain how well controlled his diabetes is based on these results.

3. What implication does the patient's issue of poor glycemic control have for his future?

→ • Click on **Return to Nurses' Station** and then on **401** to enter Harry George's room.
• Click on **Patient Care** and perform a head-to-toe assessment on the patient.

4. Below and on the next page, document any abnormal results from your assessment of Harry George.

Assessment Area	Assessment Results
Head & Neck	
Chest	
Back & Spine	

Exercise 2

CD-ROM Activity

45 minutes

• Sign in to work at Pacific View Regional Hospital for Period of Care 1. (*Note:* If you are already in the virtual hospital from a previous exercise, click on **Leave the Floor** and then **Restart the Program** to get to the sign-in window.)
• From the Patient List, select Harry George (Room 401).
• Click on **Go to Nurses' Station**.
• Click on **Chart** and then on **401**.
• Click on **History and Physical**.

1. What risk factors for diabetes are noted in Harry George's history?

2. Describe the history of this patient's present illness.

3. What is the relationship between the infection in Harry George's foot and his diabetes mellitus? (*Hint:* Read about complications of the foot on page 1123 in your textbook.)

→ • Click on **Laboratory Reports**.

4. What was Harry George's admitting blood glucose level?

5. What abnormalities in his urinalysis results can be attributed to the diabetes? Explain the relationship.

➤ • Click on **Emergency Department**.

6. What factor in Harry George's recent history most likely contributed to his hyperglycemia? (*Hint:* Read the ED physician's notes for 1345.)

➤ • Click on **Nursing Admission**.

7. Listed below are clinical manifestations of diabetes mellitus identified in the textbook. In column 2, indicate (with Yes or No) whether each manifestation is usually present in type 2 diabetes. Then indicate (with Yes or No) whether Harry George displays each manifestation based on the nurse's initial assessment.

Clinical Manifestations	Present in Type 2 DM? (Yes or No)	Experienced by Harry George? (Yes or No)
Polyuria		
Polydypsia		
Polyphagia		
Visual changes		
Weakness/fatigue		
Weight loss		
Chronic complications		
Recurrent infections		
Prolonged wound healing		

8. To what extent does Harry George fit the typical picture of a patient with type 2 diabetes mellitus?

➤ • Click on **Return to Nurses' Station** and then on **401**.
   • Select **Patient Care** and then click on **Nurse-Client Interactions**.
   • Select and view the video titled **0755: Disease Management**. (*Note:* If this video title is not available, check the virtual clock to see whether enough time has elapsed. The video cannot be viewed before its specified time.)

9. What does Harry George tell the nurse about his appetite?

10. What diet has been ordered for the patient? (*Hint:* Review his chart.)

11. Describe the principles of this diet.

12. How might the patient's alcohol intake affect his blood glucose levels?

Exercise 3

CD-ROM Activity

40 minutes

• Sign in to work at Pacific View Regional Hospital for Period of Care 2. (*Note:* If you are already in the virtual hospital from a previous exercise, click on **Leave the Floor** and then **Restart the Program** to get to the sign-in window.)
• From the Patient List, select Harry George (Room 401).
• Click on **Go to Nurses' Station**.
• Click on **Chart** and then on **401**.
• Click on **Physician's Orders**.

Assessment Area	Assessment Results
Upper Extremities	
Abdomen	
Pelvic	
Lower Extremities	

 • Click on **EPR** and **Login**. Specify **401** as the patient's room and **Neurologic** as the category.

5. List any abnormal results from the neurologic assessment on Monday at 1835.

6. Describe the potential long-term complications for DM listed below and on the next page.

Macrovascular

Diabetic retinopathy

Neuropathy

Nephropathy

7. Does Harry George exhibit signs or symptoms that would alert you to the possibility of any of the long-term complications noted in question 6? If so, explain. (*Hint:* Consider your answers to questions 4 and 5 of this exercise, as well as question 5 in Exercise 2.)

8. What patient teaching would you plan to offer this patient to prevent further injury secondary to reduced sensation in his left foot? (*Hint:* See pages 1153-1154 in your textbook.)

Diabetes Mellitus, Part 2

/Oᐆᐃᐕ **Reading Assignment:** Diabetes Mellitus and Hypoglycemia (Chapter 39)

Patient: Harry George, Room 401

Goal: Utilize the nursing process to competently administer medications prescribed to treat patients with diabetes mellitus.

Objectives:

1. Describe the pharmacologic therapy used for a patient with diabetes.
2. Evaluate a patient's response to insulin therapy.
3. Assess a patient for side effects of insulin therapy.
4. Describe the clinical manifestations of hypoglycemia as a side effect of insulin therapy.
5. Develop an individualized teaching plan for a patient with type 2 diabetes.

In this lesson you will learn the essentials regarding pharmacologic therapy for a patient admitted with complications related to diabetes mellitus. You will identify, describe, administer, and evaluate effects of prescribed antidiabetic medications. Harry George is a 54-year-old male with a 4-year history of type 2 diabetes, admitted with infection and swelling of his left foot.

Exercise 1

Clinical Preparation: Writing Activity

30 minutes

1. Identify and describe the various types of insulin by completing the table below.

Insulin Classification/ Generic Name	Brand Name	Onset (hour)	Peak (hour)	Duration (hour)
Rapid-Acting/ Aspart				
Lispro				

Insulin Classification/ Generic Name	Brand Name	Onset (hour)	Peak (hour)	Duration (hour)
Short-Acting/ Regular insulin				
Intermediate-Acting/ NPH				
Lente				
Long-Acting/ Ultralente				
Glargine				

2. Below, identify the five classifications of oral hypoglycemic agents, as well as specific medications and mechanism of action for each classification.

Classification	Medications	Mechanism of Action

Exercise 2

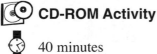

CD-ROM Activity

40 minutes

- Sign in to work at Pacific View Regional Hospital for Period of Care 1. (*Note:* If you are already in the virtual hospital from a previous exercise, click on **Leave the Floor** and then **Restart the Program** to get to the sign-in window.)
- From the Patient List, select Harry George (Room 401).
- Click on **Go to Nurses' Station**.
- Click on **Chart** and then on **401**.
- Click on **Emergency Department**.

1. What medication was ordered to control Harry George's diabetes?

2. How would you give the IV insulin? (*Hint:* Consult the Drug Guide in the Nurses' Station.)

3. Look at the ED physician's progress notes for Monday at 1345. What does the physician plan to order for the sliding scale insulin coverage?

 • Click on **Physician's Orders**.

4. Look at the orders for Monday at 1345. What was the actual sliding scale insulin order?

→ • Click on **Return to Nurses' Station**.
  • Click on **Kardex** and then on **401** for Harry George's record.

5. According to the Kardex, how often should the capillary blood glucose be tested?

→ • Click on **Return to Nurses' Station**.
  • Click on **MAR** and then on tab **401**.

6. According to the MAR, when should the insulin sliding scale be administered? What was the time of this order?

7. What would you do regarding the inconsistencies identified above?

8. What problems might you anticipate for Harry George if he does not receive insulin coverage at bedtime?

→ • Click on **Return to Nurses' Station** and then on **401** to enter Harry George's room.
  • Click on **Clinical Alerts**.

9. What is the clinical alert for 0730?

Prepare and administer the sliding scale insulin for this glucose level by following these steps:

→ • Click **Medication Room** on the bottom of the screen.
  • Click **MAR** or **Review MAR** at any time to verify how much insulin to administer based on sliding scale. (*Hint:* Remember to look at the patient name on the MAR to make sure you have the correct patient's records—you must click on correct room number within the MAR.) Click on **Return to Medication Room** after reviewing the correct MAR.

Exercise 2

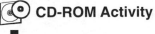 **CD-ROM Activity**

 45 minutes

- Sign in to work at Pacific View Regional Hospital for Period of Care 1. (*Note:* If you are already in the virtual hospital from a previous exercise, click on **Leave the Floor** and then **Restart the Program** to get to the sign-in window.)
- From the Patient List, select Harry George (Room 401).
- Click on **Go to Nurses' Station**.
- Click on **Chart** and then on **401**.
- Click on **History and Physical**.

1. What risk factors for diabetes are noted in Harry George's history?

2. Describe the history of this patient's present illness.

3. What is the relationship between the infection in Harry George's foot and his diabetes mellitus? (*Hint:* Read about complications of the foot on page 1123 in your textbook.)

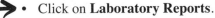 • Click on **Laboratory Reports**.

4. What was Harry George's admitting blood glucose level?

5. What abnormalities in his urinalysis results can be attributed to the diabetes? Explain the relationship.

• Click on **Emergency Department**.

6. What factor in Harry George's recent history most likely contributed to his hyperglycemia? (*Hint:* Read the ED physician's notes for 1345.)

 • Click on **Nursing Admission**.

7. Listed below are clinical manifestations of diabetes mellitus identified in the textbook. In column 2, indicate (with Yes or No) whether each manifestation is usually present in type 2 diabetes. Then indicate (with Yes or No) whether Harry George displays each manifestation based on the nurse's initial assessment.

Clinical Manifestations	Present in Type 2 DM? (Yes or No)	Experienced by Harry George? (Yes or No)
Polyuria		
Polydypsia		
Polyphagia		
Visual changes		
Weakness/fatigue		
Weight loss		
Chronic complications		
Recurrent infections		
Prolonged wound healing		

8. To what extent does Harry George fit the typical picture of a patient with type 2 diabetes mellitus?

 • Click on **Return to Nurses' Station** and then on **401**.
   • Select **Patient Care** and then click on **Nurse-Client Interactions**.
   • Select and view the video titled **0755: Disease Management**. (*Note:* If this video title is not available, check the virtual clock to see whether enough time has elapsed. The video cannot be viewed before its specified time.)

Neuropathy

Nephropathy

7. Does Harry George exhibit signs or symptoms that would alert you to the possibility of any of the long-term complications noted in question 6? If so, explain. (*Hint:* Consider your answers to questions 4 and 5 of this exercise, as well as question 5 in Exercise 2.)

 8. What patient teaching would you plan to offer this patient to prevent further injury secondary to reduced sensation in his left foot? (*Hint:* See pages 1153–1154 in your textbook.)

Assessment Area	Assessment Results
Upper Extremities	
Abdomen	
Pelvic	
Lower Extremities	

 • Click on **EPR** and **Login**. Specify **401** as the patient's room and **Neurologic** as the category.

5. List any abnormal results from the neurologic assessment on Monday at 1835.

6. Describe the potential long-term complications for DM listed below and on the next page.

Macrovascular

Diabetic retinopathy

9. What does Harry George tell the nurse about his appetite?

10. What diet has been ordered for the patient? (*Hint:* Review his chart.)

11. Describe the principles of this diet.

12. How might the patient's alcohol intake affect his blood glucose levels?

Exercise 3

CD-ROM Activity

40 minutes

- Sign in to work at Pacific View Regional Hospital for Period of Care 2. (*Note:* If you are already in the virtual hospital from a previous exercise, click on **Leave the Floor** and then **Restart the Program** to get to the sign-in window.)
- From the Patient List, select Harry George (Room 401).
- Click on **Go to Nurses' Station**.
- Click on **Chart** and then on **401**.
- Click on **Physician's Orders**.

1. What test is ordered that can be used to determine Harry George's control of diabetes mellitus? Describe the purpose of this test.

2. What was the result of this test for Harry George? Evaluate and explain how well controlled his diabetes is based on these results.

3. What implication does the patient's issue of poor glycemic control have for his future?

➤ • Click on **Return to Nurses' Station** and then on **401** to enter Harry George's room.
• Click on **Patient Care** and perform a head-to-toe assessment on the patient.

4. Below and on the next page, document any abnormal results from your assessment of Harry George.

Assessment Area	Assessment Results
Head & Neck	
Chest	
Back & Spine	

LESSON **18** _____

Nutritional Problems

_____

🕮 **Reading Assignment:** Stomach and Duodenum Problems (Chapter 42)

Patients: Harry George, Room 401
Jacquline Catanazaro, Room 402
Piya Jordan, Room 403

Goal: Utilize the nursing process to competently care for patients with nutritional disorders.

Objectives:

1. Identify patients at risk for malnutrition.
2. Perform a nutritional screening assessment on assigned patients.
3. Evaluate laboratory findings in relation to a patient's nutritional status.
4. Plan appropriate dietary interventions for a patient with malnutrition.
5. Identify a patient's risk factors related to obesity.
6. Formulate an appropriate patient education plan for an overweight patient.

In this lesson you will learn the essentials of caring for patients with nutritional disorders. You will explore each patient's history, perform a nutritional screening assessment, evaluate findings, and plan appropriate nursing interventions, including the patient's educational needs. Harry George is a 54-year-old male with a 4-year history of type 2 diabetes admitted with infection and swelling of his left foot. Piya Jordan is a 68-year-old female admitted with nausea and vomiting for several days following weeks of poor appetite and increasing weakness. Jacquline Catanazaro is a 45-year-old female admitted with an acute exacerbation of asthma.

Exercise 1

✎ **Clinical Preparation: Writing Activity**

⌚ 10 minutes

1. Describe the food guide pyramid, including the number of servings recommended for each food group. (*Hint:* Visit the FDA's website at http://www.mypyramid.gov/)

2. Below, identify the main nutrients provided by each of the five basic food groups.

Food Group	Nutrients
Bread, cereal, rice, and pasta	
Vegetables	
Fruit	
Milk, yogurt, and cheese	
Meat, poultry, fish, dry beans, eggs, nuts	

3. Record the recommended daily allowance for the following essential dietary components.

Carbohydrates

Protein

Fat

Exercise 2

 CD-Rom Activity

 40 minutes

- Sign in to work at Pacific View Regional Hospital for Period of Care 1. (*Note:* If you are already in the virtual hospital from a previous exercise, click on **Leave the Floor** and then **Restart the Program** to get to the sign-in window.)
- From the Patient List, select Harry George (Room 401) and Piya Jordan (Room 403).
- Click on **Go to Nurses' Station**.
- Click on **Chart** and then on **401** for Harry George's chart.
- Click on **History and Physical**.

1. What risk factors for malnutrition are noted in Harry George's H&P?

- Click on **Return to Nurses' Station**.
- Click on **Chart** and then on **403** for Piya Jordan's chart.
- Click on **History and Physical**.

2. What risk factors for malnutrition are noted in Piya Jordan's H&P?

- Click on **Return to Nurses' Station**.
- Click on **401** to enter Harry George's room.
- Click on **Patient Care**.

4. Calculate Harry George's body mass index (BMI) based on his current height and weight by using the following formula:

$$\frac{\text{Weight in pounds}}{\text{Height in inches x Height in inches}} \times 703 = \text{BMI}$$

 5. Evaluate the results of your findings to questions 3 and 4. What is Harry George's degree of protein depletion? (*Hint:* See pages 1230-1231 in your textbook.) Is he malnourished or at risk for malnutrition? Explain how you came to your conclusion.

Exercise 3

CD-Rom Activity

40 minutes

- Sign in to work at Pacific View Regional Hospital for Period of Care 1. (*Note:* If you are already in the virtual hospital from a previous exercise, click on **Leave the Floor** and then **Restart the Program** to get to the sign-in window.)
- From the Patient List, select Harry George (Room 401) and Piya Jordan (Room 403).
- Click on **Go to Nurses' Station**.
- Click on **403** to enter Piya Jordan's room.
- Click on **Patient Care**.

 1. Now perform the same nutritional screening assessment on Piya Jordan as you did for Harry George in the previous exercise. Referring to pages 1229-1231 in your textbook, assess the patient for any of the identified findings associated with malnutrition. Obtain subjective information by reading her History and Physical, Nursing Admission form, and laboratory results. Acquire the objective data by completing a physical assessment. Document your findings in column 3 of the table on the previous two pages.

2. Calculate Piya Jordan's BMI based on her current height and weight by using the following formula:

$$\frac{\text{Weight in pounds}}{\text{Height in inches x Height in inches}} \times 703 = \text{BMI}$$

3. Evaluate the results of your findings for questions 1 and 2. What is Piya Jordan's degree of protein depletion? (*Hint:* See pages 1230-1231 in textbook.) Is she malnourished or at risk for malnutrition? Explain how you came to your conclusion.

4. Compare and contrast your findings for Harry George and Piya Jordan. What are the similarities? What are the differences?

5. What other laboratory tests, not ordered for either of these patients, might be useful in evaluating their nutritional status?

6. Identify two nursing diagnoses related to Piya Jordan's and Harry George's malnourished status.

7. What type of diet or dietary supplements would you recommend for these two patients?

8. What additional nursing interventions would be appropriate to address these patient's nutritional needs?

Exercise 4

 CD-ROM Activity

 30 minutes

- Sign in to work at Pacific View Regional Hospital for Period of Care 2. (*Note:* If you are already in the virtual hospital from a previous exercise, click on **Leave the Floor** and then **Restart the Program** to get to the sign-in window.)
- From the Patient List, select Jacquline Catanazaro (Room 402).
- Click on **Go to Nurses' Station**.
- Click on **Chart** and then on **402**.
- Click on **Nursing Admission**.

1. Document Jacquline Catanazaro's current height and weight below.

2. Calculate her BMI using the following formula. (*Hint:* See Fig. 3.3 on page 42 in your textbook.

$$\frac{\text{Weight in pounds}}{\text{Height in inches} \times \text{Height in inches}} \times 703 = \text{BMI}$$

3. Is Jacquline Catanazaro's nutritional status normal, overweight, obese, or morbidly obese?

- Click on **History and Physical**.

4. What complication of obesity does this patient suffer from?

5. What other complications is she at risk for?

6. What are the contributing factors for Jacquline Catanazaro's increased weight?

 • Click on **Return to Nurses' Station**.
 • Click on **MAR** and then on tab **402**.

7. Do any of the medications ordered for Jacquline Catanazaro cause weight gain? If so, describe. (*Hint:* Consult the Drug Guide provided in the Nurses' Station.)

• Click on **Return to Nurses' Station**.
• Click on **402** to enter the patient's room.
• Click on **Patient Care**.
• Click on **Nurse-Client Interactions**.
• Select and view the video titled **1140: Compliance—Medications**. (*Note:* If this video title is not available, check the virtual clock to see whether enough time has elapsed. The video cannot be viewed before its specified time.)

8. What concern does the patient voice concerning her medications?

9. Evaluate the nurse's response. Was it appropriate? Accurate?

Exercise 1

Clinical Preparation: Writing Activity

20 minutes

1. Describe the pathophysiology of fluid and electrolyte imbalances associated with an intestinal obstruction.

2. Compare and contrast a mechanical and nonmechanical intestinal obstruction. (*Hint:* See page 1269 in your textbook.)

   a. Mechanical obstruction

   b. Nonmechanical obstruction

3. How does the removal of polyps help to prevent colorectal cancer? (*Hint:* Describe the relationship between polyps and cancer development.)

4. Identify the most likely site of metastasis for colorectal cancer.

Exercise 2

 CD-ROM Activity

40 minutes

- Sign in to work at Pacific View Regional Hospital for Period of Care 1. (*Note:* If you are already in the virtual hospital from a previous exercise, click on **Leave the Floor** and then **Restart the Program** to get to the sign-in window.)
- From the Patient List, select Piya Jordan (Room 403).
- Click on **Go to Nurses' Station**.
- Click on **Chart** and then on **403**.
- Click on **Emergency Department**.

1. What were Piya Jordan's presenting symptoms?

 • Click on **History and Physical**.

2. What history of symptoms is recorded?

• Click on **Laboratory Reports**.

3. Document Piya Jordan's admission electrolyte results below and on the next page. Evaluate whether each of the results is normal, decreased, or increased. Offer your rationale for any abnormalities in the last column.

	Monday 2200	Decreased, Normal, or Increased?	Rationales for Abnormality
Sodium			

	Monday 2200	Decreased, Normal, or Increased?	Rationales for Abnormality
Potassium			
Chloride			
CO_2			
Creatinine			
BUN			
Amylase			

→ • Click on **Diagnostic Reports**.

4. What was the result of the patient's KUB? What do air-fluid levels indicate?

5. Why do you think a CT scan of the abdomen was ordered? What was the result?

6. Was Piya Jordan's obstruction mechanical or nonmechanical? Explain.

7. If the patient had sought medical attention prior to the obstruction worsening, what other diagnostic testing might she have undergone? Explain what the test would show.

 • Click on **History and Physical**.

8. Now that you know Piya Jordan has a colonic mass, let's look at those presenting symptoms again. Common clinical manifestations of colorectal cancer are listed below. Place an X next to each sign or symptom consistent with the patient's history and her physical examination findings on admission.

_____ a. Rectal bleeding

_____ b. Alternating constipation and diarrhea

_____ c. Anemia

_____ d. Fatigue

_____ e. Weakness

_____ f. Colicky abdominal pain

_____ g. Vague abdominal discomfort

_____ h. Sensation of incomplete emptying

_____ i. Change in stool caliber (narrow, ribbonlike)

→ • Click on **Expired MARs**.

3. What was administered preoperatively to clean out Piya Jordan's bowel?

→ • Click on **Surgical Reports**.

4. Review the operative report. Name and describe the surgical procedure.

5. What is the most likely cell type for Piya Jordan's cancer?

6. How will the physician know what kind of cancer the tumor is?

 7. How would you classify Piya Jordan's tumor according to the Dukes' classification system? Explain. (*Hint:* See page 1276 in your textbook.)

• Click on **Laboratory Results**.

   8. Why did the physician order an amylase, lipase, and LFTs? What do the results demonstrate?

 • Click on **Return to Nurses' Station** and then on **403**.
- Click on **Patient Care** and then on **Nurse-Client Interactions**.
- Select and view the video titled **1500: Preventing Complications**. (*Note:* If this video title is not available, check the virtual clock to see whether enough time has elapsed. The video cannot be viewed before its specified time.)

   9. What nursing interventions are discussed during this brief video? Why are they appropriate for Piya Jordan?

 • Now select and view the video titled **1540: Discharge Planning**.

  10. The daughter seems to be overwhelmed by her mother's illness and needs. Describe psychosocial interventions that the nurse might plan to help the Piya Jordan and her daughter.

11. What would you teach the daughter regarding health promotion and preventing colon cancer in herself?

LESSON **20** ——————————————————

Osteomyelitis

——————————————————

📖 **Reading Assignment:** Degenerative Disorders (Chapter 53)

Patient: Harry George, Room 401

Goal: Utilize the nursing process to competently care for patients with osteomyelitis.

Objectives:

1. Describe the pathophysiology of osteomyelitis.
2. Assess an assigned patient for clinical manifestations of osteomyelitis.
3. Describe the causative agent and category of osteomyelitis in an assigned patient.
4. Safely administer IV antibiotic therapy as prescribed for osteomylelitis.
5. Evaluate diagnostic tests related to osteomyelitis.
6. Develop an individualized discharge plan of care of a patient with osteomyclitis complicated by other disease processes and homelessness.

In this lesson you will learn the essentials of caring for a patient diagnosed with osteomyelitis. You will explore the patient's history, evaluate presenting symptoms and treatment, administer prescribed medications, and develop an individualized discharge teaching plan. Harry George is a 54-year-old male admitted with infection and swelling of his left foot, a history of type 2 diabetes, alcohol abuse, and nicotine addiction.

Exercise 1

✒ **Clinical Preparation: Writing Activity**

🕐 10 minutes

1. Describe the pathophysiology of osteomyelitis.

2. Describe the two mechanisms of entry for pathogens causing osteomyelitis.

3. What is the most common causative organism of osteomyelitis?

Exercise 2

 CD-ROM Activity

35 minutes

- Sign in to work at Pacific View Regional Hospital for Period of Care 2. (*Note:* If you are already in the virtual hospital from a previous exercise, click on **Leave the Floor** and then **Restart the Program** to get to the sign-in window.)
- From the Patient List, select Harry George (Room 401).
- Click on **Go to Nurses' Station**.
- Click on **Chart** and then on **401**.
- Click on **History and Physical**.

1. The clinical manifestations of osteomyelitis can include both local and systemic symptoms. Common local and systemic signs and symptoms are listed below. Place an X next to any signs or symptoms consistent with Harry George's history and his physical examination findings on admission.

Local Symptoms	**Systemic Symptoms**
_____ Constant bone pain	_____ Fever
_____ Swelling	_____ Night sweats
_____ Tenderness	_____ Chills
_____ Warmth at infection site	_____ Restlessness
_____ Restricted movement	_____ Nausea
	_____ Malaise

2. Based on what you have read, identify the source of Harry George's osteomyelitis and the mechanism of invasion responsible for it. Explain the rationale for your conclusion.

 3. What factors in Harry George's history may have contributed to the development of osteomyelitis? (*Hint:* See pages 1589-1591 in your textbook.)

➜ • Click on **Physician's Orders**.

 4. The following diagnostic tests are useful in the diagnosis and evaluation of osteomyelitis. Match each test with its corresponding description, as given in your textbook.

Diagnostic Test	**Description**
____ MRI and CT scan	a. Initial test to determine causative organism
____ Wound culture	b. Positive in the area of infection
____ White blood cell count	c. Most definitive way to determine causative organism
____ X-ray of affected extremitiy	
____ Radionuclide bone scan	d. Elevated results of this test indicate infection
____ Bone/tissue biopsy	e. Used to help identify the extent of the infection, including soft tissue involvement
____ Erythrocyte sedimentation rate (ESR)	f. Changes with this test do not appear early in the course of the disease
	g. Elevated with inflammatory process

5. Place an X next to each diagnostic test that was performed as part of Harry George's admissions work-up.

_____ a. MRI and CT scan

_____ b. Wound culture

_____ c. White blood cell count

_____ d. X-ray of affected extremitiy

_____ e. Radionuclide bone scan

_____ f. Bone/tissue biopsy

_____ g. Erythrocyte sedimentation rate (ESR)

 • Click on **Diagnostic Reports**.

6. Compare these reports with the pathophysiology of osteomyelitis as described in the textbook. What finding is documented on these reports that is consistent with osteomyelitis? What does this finding mean?

Finding documented on the x-ray report

Finding documented on the bone scan

Meaning of both

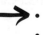 • Click on **Return to Nurses' Station**.
• Click on **MAR** and select tab **401**.

7. Determine what routine medications (excluding the continuous IV and insulin coverage) you will be giving to Harry George during the day shift (0700-1500). Below, list the medications you need to give, the drug classification, the reason why each is given, and the time each is due. (*Hint:* You may refer to the Drug Guide by returning to the Nurses' Station and clicking on the **Drug** icon in the lower left corner of your screen.)

Medication	Classification	Reason for Giving	Time Due

8. Which medication was Harry George receiving that was discontinued on Tuesday?

 • Click on **Return to Nurses' Station**.
   • Click on **Chart** and then on **401**.
   • Click on **Physician's Orders**.

9. What replaced the medication you identified in question 8?

 • Click on **Physician's Notes**.

10. Why was this change ordered?

 • Click on **Laboratory Reports**.

11. You are aware that the antibiotics have been ordered for Harry George because of his leg infection. You decide to check the WBC results because you are curious (also, you are sure your nursing instructor will ask you about it). Document the WBC results for the times specified below and indicate whether each result is normal, elevated, or decreased.

Tests	Monday 1500	Tuesday 1100	Normal, Elevated or Decreased?
Total WBC			
Neutrophil Segs			
Neutrophil Bands			
Lymphocytes			
Monocytes			
Eosinophils			
Basophils			

12. Explain what the WBC results in the table above mean, including the overall direction of the change in the WBC and the significance of this change.

→ • Click on **Return to Nurses' Station**.
• Click on **Patient List**.
• Click on **Get Report** for Harry George. Review the report.

13. Is there anything else you wish the nurse would have included in the report regarding osteomyelitis? If so, what?

→ • Click on **Return to Nurses' Station**.
• Click on **Medication Room**.
• Select **IV Storage**.
• Click on the **Small Volume** bin and choose the IV antibiotic that is due to be given at 0800.

14. What dilution of this IV antibiotic is available for you to administer?

15. Over what amount of time should you infuse the IV antibiotic? (*Hint:* You may refer to the Drug Guide for this information.)

16. If you are using an IV pump to deliver this medication piggyback, what rate (mL per hour) will you select to give this infusion?

Exercise 3

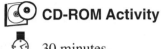 **CD-ROM Activity**

30 minutes

- Sign in to work at Pacific View Regional Hospital for Period of Care 3. (*Note:* If you are already in the virtual hospital from a previous exercise, click on **Leave the Floor** and then **Restart the Program** to get to the sign-in window.)
- From the Patient List, select Harry George (Room 401).
- Click on **Go to Nurses' Station** and then on **401**. Inside the patient's room, click on **Take Vital Signs**.

1. Record the vital sign findings below.

BP	SpO$_2$	Temp	HR	RR	Pain

 • Click on **Patient Care**.
- Click on **Lower Extremities** and complete a focused neurovascular assessment related to osteomyelitis.

2. Below, record the results of your assessment.

 • Click on **Nurse-Client Interactions**.
- Select and view the video titled **1120: Wound Management**. (*Note:* If this video title is not available, check the virtual clock to see whether enough time has elapsed. The video cannot be viewed before its specified time.)

3. How does the nurse describe the progress of Harry George's wound condition? How does the patient respond?

→ • Click on **Medication Room**.
• Click on **MAR** to determine what medications you need to administer to Harry George during this time period (1115-1200).
• Click on **Return to Medication Room**.
• Click on **IV Storage**.
• Click on the **Small Volume** bin and choose the IV antibiotic that is due to be given at 1200.
• Click **Put Medication on Tray**.
• Click on **Close Bin**.
• Click on **View Medication Room**.
• Click on **Drug** icon in the lower left corner of the screen.

4. Look up gentamicin in the Drug Guide. What must you first assess prior to administering this drug? (*Hint:* Look at alert under Administration and Handling.)

→ • Click on **Return to Medication Room**.
• Click on **Nurses' Station**.
• Click on **Chart** and then on **401**.
• Click on **Laboratory Reports**.

5. What are Harry George's most recent peak and trough levels?

6. Based on these results, what should your nursing actions be?

7. For what toxic side effects must you monitor?

8. What types of follow-up diagnostic tests should be anticipated for Harry George to determine how well the osteomyelitis is responding to therapy? What changes will occur in these diagnostic test results if therapy is effective?

9. If Harry George's infection does not respond to the antibiotic therapy, what other interventions will most likely be planned? Explain how these would benefit him.

10. Based on what you know and have read, what do you expect will be included in Harry George's discharge instructions and follow-up care to manage his osteomyelitis?

11. Based on this patient's current living conditions, how do you think his care might best be managed?

Chronic Low Back Pain

Reading Assignment: Degenerative Disorders (Chapter 53)

Patient: Jacquline Catanazaro, Room 402

Goal: Utilize the nursing process to competently care for a patient with an intervertebral disk problem.

Objectives:

1. Describe the pathophysiology of low back pain.
2. Identify clinical manifestations related to low back pain and/or herniated intervertebral disk.
3. Plan appropriate interventions to treat low back pain.
4. Evaluate a patient's potential to comply with a health care management plan.
5. Develop an individualized teaching plan for a patient with low back pain.

In this lesson you will learn the essentials of caring for a patient experiencing chronic low back pain. You will explore the patient's history, evaluate presenting symptoms and treatment, plan appropriate nursing interventions to treat the patient's symptoms, and develop an individualized discharge teaching plan. Jacquline Catanazaro is a 45-year-old female admitted with an acute exacerbation of asthma.

Exercise 1

Clinical Preparation: Writing Activity

15 minutes

1. List the risk factors for low back pain. (*Hint:* See pages 1592-1593 in your textbook.)

2. Identify five causes of low back pain.

3. Describe the pathophysiology of low back pain caused by intervertebral disc disease.

4. What differentiates acute low back pain from chronic low back pain?

5. Describe the following procedures.

   a. Laminectomy

   b. Diskectomy

   c. Microsurgical diskectomy

d. Percutaneous laser diskectomy

e. Spinal fusion

Exercise 2

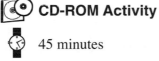 **CD-ROM Activity**

45 minutes

- Sign in to work at Pacific View Regional Hospital for Period of Care 3. (*Note:* If you are already in the virtual hospital from a previous exercise, click on **Leave the Floor** and then **Restart the Program** to get to the sign-in window.)
- From the Patient List, select Jacquline Catanazaro (Room 402).
- Click on **Go to Nurses' Station**.
- Click on **Chart** and then on **402**.
- Click on **History and Physical**.

1. Under "History of Present Illness," what are the patient's complaints related to her back?

2. How does the physician describe this problem under "Past Medical History"?

3. How was this diagnosed?

4. How long has the patient had this problem?

5. How would you classify Jacquline Catanazaro's back pain? Explain.

6. What treatment has she undergone? Explain the mechanism of action and/or rationale for these treatments.

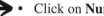 • Click on **Nursing Admission**.

7. What risk factors does Jacquline Catanazaro have for low back pain and/or herniated disc disease?

8. What assessment should be completed on this patient in relation to the back pain?

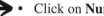 • Click on **Nurse's Notes**.

9. How have the nurses addressed Jacquline Catanazaro's complaint of low back pain?

10. What interventions could you suggest that would be appropriate for this patient's back pain during her hospital stay?

→ • Click on **History and Physical**.

 11. What is the physician's plan regarding this patient's back pain? What type of interventions might be offered by this consult? (*Hint:* See pages 1592-1593 in your textbook for interventions.)

12. According to your textbook, what intervention, noted as best clinical practice, might be helpful for Jacquline Catanazaro?

13. If her pain is not relieved by nonsurgical management, which of the procedures defined in your clinical preparation would you expect to be used for Jacquline Catanazaro? Why?

→ • Click on **Patient Education**.

14. What goals related to this patient's back pain would you add?

15. Develop a discharge teaching plan for Jacquline Catanazaro to help relieve and prevent further back pain.

→ • Click on **History and Physical**.

16. What may interfere with this patient's compliance to health care instructions?

→ • Click on **Return to Nurses' Station**.

• Click on **402** to enter Jacquline Catanazaro's room.

• Click on **Patient Care**.

• Click on **Nurse-Client Interactions**.

• Select and view the video titled **1540: Discharge Planning**. (*Note:* If this video title is not available, check the virtual clock to see whether enough time has elapsed. The video cannot be viewed before its specified time.)

17. After viewing the video, what other suggestions do you have for assisting Jacquline Catanazaro with compliance after discharge?

22

Osteoporosis

📖 **Reading Assignment:** Degenerative Disorders (Chapter 53)

Patient: Patricia Newman, Room 406

Goal: Utilize the nursing process to competently care for patients with osteoporosis.

Objectives:

1. Describe the pathophysiology of osteoporosis.
2. Assess the assigned patient for clinical manifestations of osteoporosis.
3. Describe appropriate pharmacologic therapy for prevention and/or treatment of osteo-porosis.
4. Describe the appropriate technique for safe administration of medications used to prevent or treat osteoporosis.
5. Plan appropriate interventions to promote health and prevent further bone loss in a patient with osteoporosis.
6. Develop an individualized teaching plan for an assigned patient with osteoporosis.

In this lesson you will learn the essentials of caring for a patient diagnosed with osteoporosis. You will explore the patient's history, evaluate presenting symptoms and treatment, administer prescribed medications, and develop an individualized discharge teaching plan. Patricia Newman is a 61-year-old female admitted with pneumonia and a history of emphysema.

Exercise 1

🖊 **Clinical Preparation: Writing Activity**

⏱ 10 minutes

1. Describe the pathophysiology of osteoporosis.

2. List the risk factors associated with osteoporosis. (*Hint:* See page 1588 in your textbook.)

Exercise 2

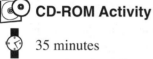 **CD-ROM Activity**

35 minutes

- Sign in to work at Pacific View Regional Hospital for Period of Care 2. (*Note:* If you are already in the virtual hospital from a previous exercise, click on **Leave the Floor** and then **Restart the Program** to get to the sign-in window.)
- From the Patient List, select Patricia Newman (Room 406).
- Click on **Go to Nurses' Station**.
- Click on **Chart** and then on **406**.
- Click on **History and Physical**.

1. How long has Patricia Newman been diagnosed with osteoporosis?

2. What risk factors does she have for osteoporosis? Are any of these modifiable? If so, which ones?

3. What diagnostic test would have been ordered to diagnose this patient's osteoporosis? Describe the test.

• Click on **Laboratory Reports**.

4. Do any laboratory results for Patricia Newman correlate with osteoporosis?

 • Click on **Nursing Admission**.

5. Are there any other risk factors found here?

6. What clinical manifestation of osteoporosis is documented on this form?

7. What other clinical manifestations would you assess Patricia Newman for in relation to osteoporosis?

 • Click on **Return to Nurses' Station**.
   • Click on **MAR** and select tab **406**.

8. What medications are ordered for Patricia Newman to help treat and prevent worsening of her osteoporosis? In the table below, identify these medications, their classifications, and mechanisms of action. You will complete the last column in question 9. (*Hint:* Consult the Drug Guide in the Nurses' Station.)

Medication	Drug Classification	Mechanism of Action	Side Effects

9. For what side effects should you monitor Patricia Newman related to these medications? Record your answer in the table above.

10. If you were to administer the prescribed estradiol to this patient, how and where would you apply it? Are there any precautions you should take while applying this?

Exercise 3

CD-ROM Activity

35 minutes

- Sign in to work at Pacific View Regional Hospital for Period of Care 3. (*Note:* If you are already in the virtual hospital from a previous exercise, click on **Leave the Floor** and then **Restart the Program** to get to the sign-in window.)
- From the Patient List, select Patricia Newman (Room 406).
- Click on **Go to Nurses' Station**.
- Click on **Chart** and then on **406**.
- Click on **Patient Education**.

1. What educational goals already identified could be related to Patricia Newman's osteoporosis?

2. What teaching would you provide her regarding exercise to prevent further bone loss?

3. What dietary needs does this patient have related to the osteoporosis? What foods would you teach her to include in her diet?

4. Complete the following table to document teaching points you would review with Patricia Newman regarding her medications to treat osteoporosis.

Medication	Teaching Points

5. If Patricia Newman asked you what further treatment might be available to her if her bone loss continued despite her present regimen, how would you answer her? (*Hint:* Identify five other drug classifications that might be useful to this patient and describe their mechanism of action.)

6. What is Patricia Newman most at risk for related to her osteoporosis?

- Click on **Return to Nurses' Station** and on **406** to enter Patricia Newman's room.
- Click on **Patient Care** and then on **Nurse-Client Education**.
- Select and view the video titled **1500: Discharge Planning**. (*Note:* If this video title is not available, check the virtual clock to see whether enough time has elapsed. The video cannot be viewed before its specified time.)

7. Although the discussion in this video was related to the patient's pulmonary disease, how would smoking cessation benefit her musculoskeletal problem?

8. What other health care disciplines might be useful to help Patricia Newman with her discharge needs related to osteoporosis?

9. What psychosocial nursing diagnosis might be a potential problem for this patient related to her slightly stooped posture and going home on oxygen? What nursing interventions would be appropriate to help her with this difficulty?

Osteoarthritis and Total Knee Replacement

⌒◯⌒ **Reading Assignment:** Osteoarthritis and Rheumatoid Arthritis (Chapter 54)

Patient: Clarence Hughes, Room 404

Goal: Utilize the nursing process to competently care for patients with osteoarthritis.

Objectives:

1. Describe clinical manifestations and treatment for a patient with debilitating osteoarthritis.
2. Document a focused assessment on a postoperative patient who has undergone a total knee arthroplasty.
3. Plan appropriate interventions to prevent complications related to a total knee replacement in an assigned patient.
4. Identify and provide rationales for collaborative care measures used to treat a patient after a total knee arthroplasty.

In this lesson you will learn the essentials of caring for a patient undergoing a total knee arthroplasty for treatment of debilitating osteoarthritis. You will document assessments, plan, implement, and evaluate care given. Clarence Hughes is a 73-year-old male admitted for an elective knee replacement. Begin this lesson by reviewing the general concepts of acid-base balance as presented in your textbook.

Exercise 1

✎ **Clinical Preparation: Writing Activity**

⌚ 10 minutes

1. Briefly describe the pathophysiology of osteoarthritis (OA).

2. List risk factors related to the occurrence of primary and/or secondary OA.

3. What are the clinical manifestations of OA?

4. What laboratory and/or radiographic testing are used in the diagnosis of OA?

Exercise 2

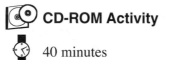 **CD-ROM Activity**

40 minutes

- Sign in to work at Pacific View Regional Hospital for Period of Care 1. (*Note:* If you are already in the virtual hospital from a previous exercise, click on **Leave the Floor** and then **Restart the Program** to get to the sign-in window.)
- From the Patient List, select Clarence Hughes (Room 404).
- Click on **Go to Nurses' Station**.
- Click on **Chart** and then on **404**.
- Click on **History and Physical**.

1. Why was Clarence Hughes admitted to the hospital?

2. Describe the symptoms that brought him to this point.

3. According to the H&P, what medications and/or treatments have been used to treat Clarence Hughes before he elected to have surgery?

 • Click on **Surgical Reports**.

4. How does the report of operation describe the surgical procedure performed on Clarence Hughes?

5. What medication was added to the cement used for this procedure? Explain the rationale for the use of this medication.

6. What was Clarence Hughes' estimated blood loss (EBL)?

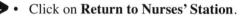

- Click on **Physician's Orders**.
- Scroll down to read the orders for Sunday 1600.

7. What frequent assessments are ordered? Describe specifically how these assessments are completed and what the nurse is looking for.

- Scroll up to read the orders for Monday 0715.

8. What is ordered for Clarence Hughes' left knee? Explain the purpose of this machine.

- Click on **Return to Nurses' Station**.
- Click on **EPR** and then on **Login**.
- Choose **404** from the Patient drop-down menu.
- Select **Intake and Output** as the category.

9. Find "Output: Drain #1" for documentation of Hemovac drainage. How much total drainage is recorded?

10. What were Clarence Hughes' I&O shift totals on Tuesday at 1500 and 2300?

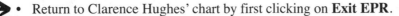

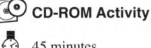
- Return to Clarence Hughes' chart by first clicking on **Exit EPR**.
- Click on **Chart** and then on **404**.
- Click on **Laboratory Reports**.

11. What was Clarence Hughes' H&H on Tuesday at 0600?

12. Why do you think his H&H was decreased? (*Hint:* Check his admitting H&H, EBL, drainage output, and 16-hour I&O on Tuesday.)

- Click on **Physician's Orders**.

13. What was ordered to correct the above laboratory result?

Exercise 3

CD-ROM Activity

45 minutes

- Sign in to work at Pacific View Regional Hospital for Period of Care 1. (*Note:* If you are already in the virtual hospital from a previous exercise, click on **Leave the Floor** and then **Restart the Program** to get to the sign-in window.)
- From the Patient List, select Clarence Hughes (Room 404).
- Click on **Get Report**.

1. What are your concerns for Clarence Hughes after receiving report?

→ • Click on **Go to Nurses' Station**.
  • Click on **404** to go to the patient's room.
  • Click on **Patient Care**.

2. Based on Clarence Hughes' diagnosis and surgery, complete a focused assessment and document your findings below.

Area Assessed	Findings
a.	
b.	
c.	
d.	
e.	

→ • Click on **Clinical Alerts**.

   3. Based on these findings what would be your priority interventions?

→ • Click on **Medication Room**.

   • Click on **MAR** to determine prn medications that have been ordered for Clarence Hughes to address his constipation and pain. (*Note:* You may click on **Review MAR** at any time to verify correct medication order. Remember to look at the patient name on the MAR to make sure you have the correct patient's record—you must click on the correct room number within the MAR. Click on **Return to Medication Room** after reviewing the correct MAR.)

   • Click on **Unit Dosage** (or on the Unit Dosage cabinet); from the close-up view, click on drawer **404**.

   • Select the medications you would like to administer. After each selection, click **Put Medication on Tray**. When you are finished selecting medications, click **Close Drawer**.

   • Click on **View Medication Room**.

   • Click on **Automated System** (or on the Automated System unit itself). Click **Login**.

   • On the next screen, specify the correct patient and drawer location.

   • Select the medication you would like to administer and click on **Put Medication on Tray**. Repeat this process if you wish to administer other medications from the Automated System.

   • When you are finished, click **Close Drawer**. At the bottom right corner of the next screen, click on **View Medication Room**.

   • From the Medication Room, click on **Preparation** (or on the preparation tray).

   • From the list of medications on your tray, choose the correct medication to administer.

   • Click **Next**, specify the correct patient to administer this medication to, and click **Finish**.

   • Repeat the previous two steps until all medications that you want to administer are prepared.

   • You can click on **Review Your Medications** and then on **Return to Medication Room** when ready. Once you are back in the Medication Room, you may go directly to Clarence Hughes' room by clicking on **404** at bottom of screen.

   • Administer the medication, utilizing the five rights of medication administration. After you have collected the appropriate assessment data and are ready for administration, click **Patient Care** and then **Medication Administration**. Verify that the correct patient and medication(s) appear in the left-hand window. Then click the down arrow next to Select. From the drop-down menu, select **Administer** and complete the Administration Wizard by providing any information requested. When the Wizard stops asking for information, click **Administer to Patient**. Specify **Yes** when asked whether this administration should be recorded in the MAR. Finally, click **Finish**. You will evaluate your performance in this area at the end of this exercise (see question 14).

   4. What is missing on the patient's order for oxycodone with acetaminophen? What measures need to be taken?

5. Based on the knowledge that most antacids frequently decrease absorption of other medications when concurrently administered, what options might the nurse employ to ensure adequate absorption of pain medication? (*Hint:* Consult the Drug Guide.)

 • Still in Clarence Hughes' room, click on **Nurse-Client Interactions**. (*Hint:* If this selection is not available, click first on **Patient Care** to access the additional options.)

• Select and view the video titled **0735: Empathy**. (*Note:* If this video title is not available, check the virtual clock to see whether enough time has elapsed. The video cannot be viewed before its specified time.)

6. The nurse attempts to appear empathetic by offering to listen to the patient's concerns. Are her actions congruent with her verbal communication? Why or why not?

7. If you were Clarence Hughes' nurse, what would you do differently?

8. While planning nursing care for Clarence Hughes, identify potential complications related to his postoperative status and measures that can be employed to prevent them. Document your plan of care below.

Complications   **Preventative Measures**

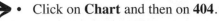 • Click on **Chart** and then on **404**.
- Click on **Consultations**.

9. What is physical therapy (PT) doing for Clarence Hughes?

 • Click on **Physician's Orders**.

10. What is the patient's activity order for Wednesday morning?

 • Click on **Nurse's Notes**.

11. What is the patient's goal for CPM therapy today?

12. Do you think the ambulation and CPM goals are sufficient for the patient to be discharged tomorrow? Why or why not? (*Hint:* Look at home situation in nursing admission form.)

 • Click on **Patient Education**.

13. What teaching should be completed for Clarence Hughes before his discharge?

Now let's see how you did during your earlier medication administration!

→ • Click on **Leave the Floor** at the bottom of your screen. From the Floor Menu, select **Look at Your Preceptor's Evaluation**. Then click on **Medication Scorecard**.

14. Disregard the report for the routine scheduled medications but note below whether or not you correctly administered the appropriate prn medications. If not, why do you think you were incorrect? According to Table C in this scorecard, what resources should be used and what important assessments should be completed before administering these medications? Did you utilize these resources and perform these assessments correctly?

LESSON 24 ———————————————————————

Glaucoma

———————————————————————

Reading Assignment: Problems of the Eye (Chapter 61)

Patient: Clarence Hughes, Room 404

Goal: Utilize the nursing process to competently care for patients with glaucoma.

Objectives:

1. Describe the pathophysiology of glaucoma.
2. Identify clinical manifestations related to glaucoma.
3. Describe appropriate pharmacologic treatment of glaucoma.
4. Administer eyedrops safely and accurately.
5. Evaluate a patient's ability to correctly administer prescribed ophthalmic medication.

In this lesson you will learn the essentials of caring for a patient diagnosed with glaucoma. You will explore the patient's history, evaluate presenting symptoms and treatment, administer prescribed medications, and develop an individualized discharge teaching plan. Clarence Hughes is a 73-year-old man admitted for an elective left knee arthroplasty.

Exercise 1

Clinical Preparation: Writing Activity

15 minutes

1. Briefly describe the general pathophysiology of glaucoma.

2. Compare and contrast the three different types of glaucoma by completing the following table.

Type of Glaucoma	Etiology	Pathophysiology	Clinical Manifestions
Primary open-angle			
Primary angle-closure			
Secondary			

 3. What measures are used to diagnose glaucoma? (*Hint:* See page 1819 in your textbook.)

Exercise 2

 CD-ROM Activity

45 minutes

- Sign in to work at Pacific View Regional Hospital for Period of Care 3. (*Note:* If you are already in the virtual hospital from a previous exercise, click on **Leave the Floor** and then **Restart the Program** to get to the sign-in window.)
- From the Patient List, select Clarence Hughes (Room 404).
- Click on **Go to Nurses' Station**.
- Click on **Chart** and then on **404**.
- Click on **History and Physical**.

1. What problems of the eye does Clarence Hughes have?

2. How would this be diagnosed?

3. What signs and symptoms do you think he had prior to diagnosis?

4. What clinical manifestation(s) should you now assess for related to this diagnosis?

5. The H&P does not identify the type of glaucoma Clarence Hughes has. Based on his history and information in the textbook, which type do you think he mostly likely has? Explain why you came to this conclusion. (*Hint:* See page 1818-1819 in your textbook.)

→ • Click on **Return to Nurses' Station**.
   • Click on **MAR** and then on tab **404**.

6. What medications are ordered for Clarence Hughes' glaucoma? Identify these medications, their classifications, and mechanisms of action below. (*Note:* You will complete the last column in question 7.)

Medication	Drug Classification	Mechanism of Action	Side Effects

7. For what side effects should you monitor Clarence Hughes related to these medications? Record your answer in the table above.

8. If you were to administer the prescribed antiglaucoma medication to Clarence Hughes, how would you correctly apply the eye drops? Explain the step-by-step procedure. (*Hint:* Consult the Drug Guide by clicking on the **Drug** icon in the lower left corner of your screen.)

9. What range of IOP would Clarence Hughes have had prior to beginning treatment for glaucoma? What would you expect his reading to be during treatment?

→ • Click on **Return to Nurses' Station**.
  • Click on **Chart** and then on **404**.
  • Click on **Patient Education**.

10. What educational goals would you add for Clarence Hughes related to his glaucoma?

11. What teaching would you provide this patient regarding his glaucoma?

12. Complete the following table by documenting teaching points you would review with Clarence Hughes regarding his glaucoma medications.

Medication	Teaching Points

13. What teaching methods would you use to teach medication administration to this patient?

14. How would you evaluate Clarence Hughes' understanding of correct medication application?

15. If Clarence Hughes' ophthalmic medications would fail to maintain IOP within normal limits, what other therapy might he expect to undergo? Briefly describe each procedure.

Notes:

Notes: